QUICK
HEADACHE
RELIEF
WITHOUT
DRUGS

Quick Headache Relief Without Drugs

HOWARD KURLAND, M.D.

ORBIS PUBLISHING LIMITED
London

I wish to express my gratitude and appreciation to Max Gunther for his skillful collaboration in the preparation of this book.

CONTENTS

CONTENTS

LIST OF
ILLUSTRATIONS

HOWARD D. KURLAND, M.D., is Professor, Department of Psychiatry at Northwestern University Medical School, past President of the Association for General Hospital Psychiatry, former Chief of Psychiatric Service of the Veterans Administration Research Hospital in Chicago, Senior Attending Psychiatrist and Senior Attending Neurologist at Evanston Hospital, Evanston, Illinois, and President of the Board of Directors of the National Board of Acupuncture Medicine, Inc.

AUTO-ACUPRESSURE has rescued many of my patients from a lifetime of drug-taking. The main reason for writing this book is my hope that it will rescue many other headache sufferers from the same fate. The technique has worked for people who had been taking much more than an occasional handful of aspirins. Some of my patients were ingesting so many powerful drugs that it was hard to see how they could carry on normal daily lives. They were, in truth, prisoners of pain—and of pain-relieving drugs. If you are one of these prisoners, and certainly if your headache problems are less serious, this book, carefully read and properly applied, will help you to free yourself.

H.D.K.

QUICK
HEADACHE
RELIEF
WITHOUT
DRUGS

**PAINS,
PILLS,
AND
PRESSURE**

HEADACHE. Of all kinds of pain that afflict mankind, it may be the most common. It is also, unfortunately, a kind of pain for which the typical sufferer has never found a really satisfactory treatment. Up to now. And I do not add those three words carelessly.

I assume you have picked up this book because you are only too well acquainted with headaches. At least ninety percent of adults are so afflicted to some degree. Some headaches are mild enough to be little more than a nuisance, while others are so severe as to be incapacitating. Some people's headaches come rarely and last less than a day, while other people suffer almost constantly. But whether mild or severe, hours long or weeks long, rare or chronic, headaches bring a kind of misery that everyone would rather be without. At its mildest, a headache takes the joy out of life. It lowers your efficiency in work and play. It changes your personality. Where once you were happy, you become a grouch; where once serene, you are irritable and jumpy and easily upset. You are no fun for others to be with, and you are no fun for yourself, either.

What is the answer? For most sufferers, pain-killing drugs. Most likely you buy these for yourself from a drugstore or supermarket. Enormous quantities of analgesics are sold without prescription in this country and in Europe. Acetylsalicylic acid, sold in the form of aspirin tablets, and also an ingredient in many combination drugs, such as Anacin and Bufferin, is produced in the United States at a rate of eighty thousand to one hundred thousand pounds *a day*.

If your pain has been more severe or intractable than average, perhaps you have a medical doctor's prescription for some more powerful drug. But whether you depend on prescription medicines or over-the-counter products, or both, you may often have asked yourself whether all these alien chemicals so casually and frequently poured into your body are doing you any good.

The question is well worth asking, and asking seriously. For the answer is almost certainly *no*: Those drugs are not doing you any good except (when they work) to give you transitory relief from the ache in your head.

There are unwanted short-term side effects that you have undoubtedly noticed. When you have been drugged, even by relatively mild pain relievers, your body is unavoidably operating at less than peak efficiency. You feel dull or woozy, perhaps. You plod through the day mechanically, unable to concentrate, missing much. Life's bright colors grow dim—"as though I'm walking around wrapped in some kind of gray fog," a patient once complained to me.

There are also side effects of the utmost seriousness—effects that, even with those supposedly "mild" nonprescription drugs you buy at the supermarket, can lead to severe illness and even death. Probably the most dramatic of these effects is death by overdose. Of all such deaths in the United States each year, the second leading cause (the first being barbiturates) is aspirin.

Other effects, though perhaps less dramatic, can be equally serious. Aspirin, the most commonly used nonprescription drug, causes gastric irritation. In many people, a normal ten-grain dose (two tablets) may cause about a teaspoon of blood to be lost through the delicate inner lining of the stomach. If this irritation continues over a span of time, it may lead to peptic ulceration. Components of other common over-the-counter headache remedies—phenacetin, for example—have their own toxic, and sometimes deadly, effects.

There are unwanted and often dangerous side effects with prescription drugs, too. Strong pain admittedly requires strong medicine. If a patient is suffering from severe, disabling headaches, such as migraine, a physician may prescribe a potentially dangerous drug on the basis that it is the lesser of two evils. He and

QUICK HEADACHE RELIEF
WITHOUT DRUGS

the patient must make a hard choice: the pain or the danger. If the patient's agony is so intolerable that it seriously interferes with normal living, there may seem to be no real choice at all. The danger simply has to be accepted as part of the bargain.

It would be nice if there were a third choice. I am writing this book to tell you that there is.

Auto-acupressure is a medical technique by which you can reduce or eliminate your own headaches without drugs. The basis of the technique is pressure, applied in a certain way at specific points on your body. The technique is a modification of acupuncture, in which pain or other problems are treated by inserting and manipulating needles at certain carefully chosen body points. The acupressure technique, however, requires no needles. All you need are your own two thumbs.

In the past three years I have treated several hundred headache sufferers with acupressure, showing them the self-treatment technique that I'm going to teach you. Some of these men and women were patients at Evanston Hospital, where I have been a Senior Attending Neurologist and Psychiatrist. Others were people who had consulted me in my private office. At medical meetings I have demonstrated the technique to so many other men and women that I've lost count.

With the majority of people suffering from migraine and other common headaches, acupressure, when properly applied, makes the pain diminish appreciably or disappear altogether almost instantly. Some need to give themselves repeat treatments, just as you sometimes need repeat doses or bigger-than-usual doses of a pain-deadening drug. But with auto-acupressure, unlike drugs, it is impossible to "overdose." Some report that the headache does not always go away entirely but becomes tolerable, or lasts for a shorter time than the headaches they have known in the past. A *very* small minority seem not to be helped (apparently, in some cases, because they are not willing to apply the pressure forcefully enough).

There are people who get little or no headache relief from pain-killing drugs in normal doses and they have to keep stepping up the dosage to dangerous levels. This is one of the major difficulties with drug-taking. There is a limit to the amount of aspirin or Anacin or Excedrin you can take safely in a day. There is no limit, however, as I have pointed out, to the number of auto-acupressure treatments you can give yourself in a day. If you find you are one of those people who do not get full or lasting relief from one treatment, you can give yourself another with perfect safety, no matter how much or little time has elapsed since your last treatment.

* * *

QUICK HEADACHE RELIEF
WITHOUT DRUGS

I am keenly aware that I have a wall of skepticism to climb before I can convince you and others that the technique really works. My own initial skepticism was greater than any I have encountered, so I am hardly in a position to object to the skepticism of others. In fact, I welcome it, especially when it comes from my colleagues in the medical profession. No newly proposed medical treatment should ever be accepted uncritically. There must always be a prologue of honest skepticism, a period of careful evaluation and even profound doubt. At this particular point in our cultural history, this skepticism is doubly necessary in the case of any treatment related to acupuncture. That includes auto-acupressure, which is sometimes referred to as "acupuncture without needles."

Acupuncture, unfortunately, has become something of a fad in America during the past several years. Too many people have embraced it too uncritically. Promises have been made that have not been kept. Hopes have been raised only to be dashed. Acupuncture has been used indiscriminately to treat diseases that are not amenable to it, and it has been used by an astounding collection of people from serious medical practitioners to wild-eyed mystics to blunderers to plain, old-fashioned quacks. As a result, many people think it is all nonsense. This is unfortunate—and I will make some more comments on this situation later.

Behind this growing awareness that acupuncture

lacks the magic cure-all properties for which some once hailed it, there lies a deeper and more philosophical problem. Acupuncture is associated in many people's minds with Oriental mysticism. Since the middle 1960s or thereabouts, certain segments of the population—notably younger men and women—have looked to the East in a hopeful search for tranquillity or some other quality of life that they feel is lacking in our modern, industrial, urban Western culture. For some, the Indian or Tibetan guru (or the man claiming to be one) has replaced the Western-style psychiatrist or church minister. That segment of the population has embraced the mystic philosophies of the East and has loudly applauded them as the answer to all our very painful troubles. Another segment, much larger, has denounced the Eastward-reaching movement as self-delusive at best and a sorry sham at worst—a wishful attempt to escape real-life problems instead of facing them and solving them.

Acupuncture, sadly, has been caught up in this cultural quarrel. Those who automatically embrace everything Oriental will naturally embrace acupuncture, too—often without studying it carefully and, just as often, surrounding it with Eastern mystical trappings that do not really have anything to do with it. Those who reject the Eastward-reaching movement will often reject acupuncture as part of it, again without study.

Thus, I must deal with two kinds of skepticism:

QUICK HEADACHE RELIEF
WITHOUT DRUGS

---

the kind that should always greet a newly proposed
medical treatment of any sort, plus the kind that now
greets anything with an Oriental-mystical sound. As I
remarked before, skepticism does not trouble me. Indeed, I would have been greatly disappointed in my
medical colleagues if they had *failed* to show skepticism.

They have not disappointed me. I had to work
hard to dispel doubt among residents at the Northwestern University Medical School, where I teach. I
also had to work hard at a recent (1975) California
meeting of the American Psychiatric Association,
where I presented a paper on my acupressure technique.

After my presentation, I offered to relieve the
headache of anybody in the audience who happened
to be suffering at the moment. About a dozen people
came up to the podium to avail themselves of the offer.
I treated the dozen volunteers, all of them M.D.s, and
many of them psychiatrists. To the surprise of the
more skeptical ones, their headaches were relieved on
the spot.

One of the most skeptical was a psychiatrist who
proclaimed loudly that I was practicing a form of
hypnosis. Another thought perhaps he could achieve
the same results. He watched me work on my "patients"
for a while, then said he would like to try. On the
next volunteer, he pressed roughly where he had seen
me press.

He did not press in the right way or on exactly the right areas, however. The "hypnosis" failed to work, and the subject announced that his headache was still with him. I went to him and pressed in the right places. The man smiled, nodded, and announced that his headache was gone.

Auto-acupressure has rescued many of my patients from a lifetime of drug-taking. The main reason for writing this book is my hope that it will rescue a lot of other headache sufferers from the same fate. The technique has worked for people who had been taking much more than an occasional handful of aspirins. Some of my patients were ingesting so many powerful drugs that it was hard to see how they could carry on normal daily lives. They were, in truth, prisoners of pain—and of pain-relieving drugs.

One thirty-eight-year-old man came to me with a history of intolerable migraine headaches going back to his boyhood. His headaches were of the kind called histamine cephalgia, generally the worst kind of migraine. For about a decade and a half, the headaches had occurred in clusters spanning roughly a week each. They often started in his sleep. He would wake up suddenly with a fierce, penetrating, throbbing pain in one side of his head. He would find himself drenched with sweat. There was extreme nausea with most of the attacks, and in some of the worst ones his vision was affected. The pain and associated symptoms were so severe that he was often unable to function at all during an attack. "I can't work, can't think, can't even eat a lot of the time," he told me miserably. While in the midst of a cluster of these attacks he had little choice but to lie in bed, get up occasionally when the pain subsided, and fall back into bed when a new bout of those agonizing symptoms struck.

He had consulted neurologists and had been given prescriptions for many kinds of drugs. He had tried migraine preventives, such as Sansert, and treatment agents, such as antihistamines (e.g., Benadryl) and ergotamine (e.g., Cafergot). For the pain, he had used codeine and Darvon. Though these medicines reduced the intensity of many individual attacks, they were of little use for migraines that woke him in the middle of the night. He could not casually take such strong drugs before he went to sleep each night, on the chance that a new headache cluster was on the way. The medicines were expensive and also—as he had been warned—dangerous if taken in too large a quantity. To supplement his normal dose of prescription drugs he had swallowed huge amounts of over-the-counter analgesics, such as aspirin and Tylenol.

This was how I first saw him: a man living in constant fear of disabling pain, sentenced to a drug-taking life-style and understandably in despair about it.

After a thorough medical evaluation to make sure

no serious illness or injury was causing or contributing to the pain, I gave the man three acupuncture treatments. I administered each treatment at a time when a severe headache was actually under way. My main purpose in doing this was to find out whether these unusually severe headaches would respond well to this kind of treatment. The answer was yes. The man's pain and nausea were significantly lessened each time.

Then I told him it probably would not be necessary for him to come back to me every time a new cluster of headaches descended on him. He could treat the headaches himself, using thumb pressure in the manner I demonstrated to him and will demonstrate to you in this book. I gave him instructions on exactly where and how to apply the pressure, and then sent him on his way.

It worked out as I had hoped. In a month or so he was able to stop using the ergotamine (Cafergot) preparations, Sansert, antihistamines, codeine, and Darvon. Within a year he had almost stopped using over-the-counter pain pills, too. When I saw him at the end of two years, he told me that his total use of drugs during the past year had been three doses of Tylenol: six tablets in twelve months!

His headaches had not vanished completely. It is rare that headaches of such massive intensity that have lasted most of a lifetime can be switched off the way you might switch off a loud radio that is annoying you—

rare no matter what the treatment. But the improvement was remarkable, all the difference between a life of intense pain or dread of pain and a virtually normal existence.

Now my patient's headache clusters came less often, and each cluster lasted only two days instead of a week. Within each cluster, he was able to alleviate each new spear of pain by quickly applying acupressure. One of his problems in the past had been that the pain spasms sometimes occurred within minutes of each other, and the only way to tolerate the agony was to keep himself drugged into a half-dazed state for days at a time. Using acupressure, he could attack each spasm directly as it hit him, whether at night or in the middle of a working day. The pain and nausea were virtually eliminated. He had won his life back.

Another patient, a fifty-year-old woman, was afflicted with such unbearable pain that the thought of giving up pain medications literally terrified her. "I can't do it, I just don't have the courage," she told me in a voice that had real fear in it. "You don't know what these headaches are like! I couldn't face them without something to kill the pain."

I could readily sympathize with her. From her point of view, that overwhelming fear was well justified. Her headaches came often, lasted several days, and were characterized by a crushing, throbbing pain in the front of the head. Strong prescription pain medications relieved the agony only partially, and even when heavily drugged she had to spend most of the headache's duration in bed.

There were special medical considerations in her case. She had diabetes of a kind that was not easy to control. She was in the care of a physician who specialized in that disease, and she always followed his instructions carefully. Despite his and her best efforts, there were periods when her blood sugar dropped too low. This condition, called hypoglycemia, is known to bring on headaches for many people, as it did with her.

I told her never to ignore the symptoms of hypoglycemia. Merely treating the headache while ignoring the low blood sugar condition itself could be highly dangerous. Whenever she noticed those symptoms, she was to go to her specialist immediately. Meanwhile, I taught her auto-acupressure to alleviate the headaches.

She made little progress at first. The headaches were so severe and her fear of them so great that she could not imagine living without her supply of narcotics. Even when auto-acupressure cut down both the frequency and the severity of the headaches, she clung desperately to the drugs that had been her only escape from torment.

But then, toward the end of the first year, she seemed to grow more skillful in using the technique. Perhaps she had not trusted it before. Perhaps she had not tried hard enough. Whatever the reason, she began to find that the pressure treatments were giving her even more complete and long-lasting relief from pain. Little by little, she liberated herself from dependence on narcotics. She has eliminated them completely for the past two years.

The man and the woman in these two cases were afflicted with unusually severe chronic headaches: misery so intense and intractable that normal living was impossible. The majority of headache victims, though, suffer much less. If you are in that lucky majority (I use the word *lucky* in a relative sense, of course), you probably do not think of headache as a disabling illness. Perhaps once in a while you are hit by a headache that lands you in bed, but more often you are one of the walking wounded. You tell yourself, "I *won't* let it keep me down," and you swallow handfuls of pills and stumble through your daily obligations.

Wouldn't life be better if you could attack the headaches without the pills?

CHAPTER

2

A WORD
TO
THE SKEPTICS

MANY OF MY PATIENTS have been startled when I first suggested using auto-acupressure to relieve headaches. Most have been skeptical.

This is perfectly understandable. In our society, people are taught from childhood that the way to attack headaches is to take pills. It becomes almost a reflex action: If your head hurts, you reach for the pill bottle. One dangerous feature of pills is the fact that they do usually work for people whose headaches are relatively mild and infrequent. The damage done by these medicines may be hidden and may take years or decades to develop into a serious problem. Meanwhile, for many people, the pills go on relieving head pain effectively enough. Each time this relief occurs, the headache sufferer's faith in pills is reinforced. The sufferer is not aware of the potentially serious damage being wrought inside his or her body by those seemingly harmless chemicals. If there are any tangible after-effects, they are usually fairly trivial and of short duration. The sufferer is aware of only one thing: Another headache has been relieved.

People with unusually acute headaches, the kind

that cannot be relieved by conventional over-the-counter medicines, are often more ready to listen when I start talking about auto-acupressure. Many of these people are desperate. They may have been taking strong prescription drugs whose side effects are tangible and often alarming. They may be ready to try almost anything that will help them escape the drug-taking life-style. But people with what might be called "ordinary" headaches are sometimes harder to convince. The typical man or woman who experiences occasional migraine or tension headaches—headaches that are not usually incapacitating and may be little more than a periodic nuisance—may feel there is little reason to stop buying pain-relieving drugs.

"Aspirin always seemed to work fine for me," one woman patient recalled. "My mother and grandmother used to take aspirin for headaches, and my grandfather used to take huge amounts for arthritis pain in his knees. We always had aspirin around the house. My mother would no more think of running out of aspirin than running out of bread. She didn't know it was a potentially dangerous drug and neither did anybody else, as far as I can recall. It was something that every household had to have. I remember taking it even when I was a small child. My mother gave it to me for almost any complaint—a headache, a cold, a sprained ankle. Aspirin and a glass of milk. That was her pet remedy for just about everything."

Thus does our society encourage a pill-taking attitude toward life. As the woman so accurately describes it, pills even become part of mothering. A mother expresses love and sympathy by giving a child a pill.

This particular woman—I will call her Jeanette T. —suffered from occasional migraines. Like most people, she considered them one of life's unavoidable irritations —"like mosquitoes and inflation," as she put it. They were not the agonizing, incapacitating kind that prevent normal functioning. As a matter of fact—again like most people—she had never consulted a physician about them. She had come to me for other reasons and mentioned the headaches as a peripheral issue. However, I was concerned about her too-casual use of analgesics and tried to encourage her to use auto-acupressure instead.

Jeanette was dubious. "I tried acupressure the next few times I had a headache," she recalled later. "It seemed to work all right, but I guess I didn't really trust it. I kept thinking the headache would come back, so I took aspirin just to be sure. I didn't give acupressure a fair test. After all, when you've been taking pills since childhood, it's hard to get out of the habit."

Then a day came when she found herself with a headache but without access to her pills. She was on board a train, with a two-hour trip ahead of her. "I'd felt a headache coming on for about an hour before getting on the train, but I'd been so rushed that there wasn't any time to stop and take aspirin. I planned to take some pills on the train. But when I looked in my bag, I found I didn't have them with me. The headache was a bad one. There was nothing to do but try acupressure."

I had taught her some special techniques for applying auto-acupressure that would be inconspicuous if she was in a public place, techniques that I will teach you later in the book. She sat there in her seat on the train and treated herself carefully and well for the first time. "I was still skeptical, still wishing I had some aspirin. I told myself, 'Well, it'll be all right, I'll buy some aspirin when I get off the train.' When I finished with the acupressure, the headache was definitely diminished, but I expected it to come back. I picked up a magazine and started to read. Then, about twenty minutes later, I suddenly looked up from the magazine and realized that the headache was gone entirely. I never did buy the aspirin. I've hardly ever used any since."

Another skeptical patient, a man whom I'll call Fred C., was also a victim of "ordinary" headaches. His were not migraines but were a combination of what a layman might term "tension" and "hunger" headaches. He was an on-the-road salesman. On days when he felt rushed and tense, subsisting on snacks instead of meals, he often found his head hurting by evening. With him, as with Jeanette, headaches were not a major problem in his life, but he certainly did not enjoy them when they arrived and would have been happy to banish them if he could.

A Word to the Skeptics

His problem was that he had read a book on Shiatsu, a Japanese thumb-pressure technique. He had not been impressed. The book had presented Shiatsu self-treatments as a means of relieving many different ailments—not only headaches but also decreased sexual vigor, insomnia, constipation, and many others. Fred commented sourly that it all sounded like quackery to him. And so he was skeptical about auto-acupressure, which also uses the thumbs.

I told him that Shiatsu is practiced in Japan by trained masseurs. It is not intended to replace medical treatment but to supplement it. No single treatment can be effective for all diseases. I have read many books on Shiatsu; however, none of them have recommended treating headaches by stimulating the areas that will be described in this book.

Shiatsu and acupressure are both related to acupuncture. All three treatment methods depend on stimulating certain nerves in various rigidly prescribed ways. Acupuncture, of course, achieves this stimulation by insertion of needles. In this sense it is the most accurate of the three, the most delicately controllable. If you are aiming for a certain small point on a nerve pathway, obviously you can stimulate that point more precisely with a needle than with anything else.

Shiatsu practitioners, instead, often use the pads of the thumbs, applying thumb pressure as the extension of total body weight and strength. They deal with some of the same nerve-stimulation points as does acupuncture, but the stimulation they apply is more diffuse—spread over the entire area of the thumb pad or base of the palm of the hand rather than being concentrated at the point of a needle. In order to achieve the necessary degree of stimulation on a nerve, they must use enormous force. Professional Shiatsu practitioners and Chinese acupuncturists specializing in massage often have visibly overdeveloped thumb joints. In the Orient, I have seen such masseurs produce bruises on their patients.

If that much force is necessary, it seems overoptimistic to assume that a novice, getting instructions from a book, could do an effective treatment job on himself or herself. My system of auto-acupressure requires much less force. Instead of using the thumb pads or palms, it uses the *thumbnails.* Thus, though it is less of a precision instrument than stimulation by a needle, it comes closer to its effectiveness. Auto-acupressure produces a degree of pressure that is much less diffuse than that of Shiatsu. Some force is required, but no more than any man or woman can apply easily, without long training.

Moreover, as I told Fred C. and as I will stress in this book, I do not offer auto-acupressure as a remedy for many diverse ills. Acupuncture techniques cannot replace your medical doctor. Moreover, professional acupuncturists and Shiatsu practitioners spend years learning to locate and stimulate nerve points with precision. There are hundreds of points on the body, each purportedly related to a different medical problem. In this book I will concentrate exclusively on the use of auto-acupressure for relieving headache pain. As you will discover, even this narrowly limited subject cannot be learned casually overnight. Effective auto-acupressure requires knowledge and practice. There are not a great many pressure points for you to locate on your body, but you *must* locate them with precision and learn to press them in exactly the right ways. If you do not, the treatment will be ineffective.

Fred C. went away and thought about what I had said. Like Jeanette T., he was not willing to abandon a nearly lifelong habit of taking over-the-counter drugs to relieve his headaches. As he reported later, "I used auto-acupressure once in a while but I never let my pill bottle get too far away." Instead of taking aspirin, he usually preferred another popular drug whose manufacturer advertised that it did not upset the stomach like aspirin. On days when headaches were troubling him, he would take six or eight of the pills in a twenty-four-hour period.

"The big change for me," he recalled, "came at the end of a really frantic week. It was one of those weeks when I always had to be in two places at once, with a new emergency every half hour, people yelling at me, nothing going right. By the middle of each day I'd have a headache. I was taking pills every time I could get near a glass of water. Around the end of the week, maybe Thursday, I not only had a headache but an upset stomach too. The worst of it was that I kept tasting those pills. I guess my stomach didn't want them and was trying to tell me so. But I kept on swallowing them all the rest of that day because my headache was so bad.

"I woke up the next morning with that taste still in my mouth. I felt awful; the indigestion was so bad that I didn't even want breakfast. Around midmorning the headache started to come back. I got out a couple of pills, looked at them, and suddenly said to myself, 'No, I *don't* want them. I'd rather live with the headache.' Then I had a new thought: 'I'll try acupressure.' I did it carefully this time, because I was determined not to take any more pills. I don't think I really expected it to work—but it did. As a matter of fact, it worked much faster than the pills ever had."

Your experience, when you begin using auto-acupressure, may be similar. Even though you may not feel as closely wedded to pills as Jeanette and Fred did, the unfortunate fact is that you are living in a culture that overemphasizes drugs. It may take a certain effort of will on your part to put acupressure to a fair test. But I am virtually certain that, once you have done that, you will feel less need for headache drugs than you once did. Perhaps, indeed, you will have no further need for them at all.

CHAPTER

3

THE LONG
JOURNEY EAST
OF A
WESTERN
PHYSICIAN

IF I HOPE to convince you that auto-acupressure is medically sound, I think I had better begin by telling you how I was convinced.

It was not easy. I recall visiting a friend in Hong Kong many years ago. He and I spent a delightful day sailing around the harbor on his boat. During the day we talked much about the East and West: the differences in philosophy, social forms, attitudes toward life and death. One subject we debated passionately was acupuncture.

Living in the Orient, he had learned about acupuncture. He had watched it performed and believed it was a useful medical procedure. As a Western-trained and specifically an American-trained physician, I doubted it was useful. I could not comprehend why it should be.

My friend told me stories of people he knew who felt that acupuncture had helped them get rid of various ills and aches. There was no reason to think he was lying to me. The stories, as he had heard them, may have been true. Rather than arguing about the stories themselves, I was forced into the position of arguing about the rationale.

"All right," I said, "I'll grant that there are people who think acupuncture cured them of this and that. But there could be all kinds of explanations. In a lot of cases, the patient was going to get better anyway. The patient credits acupuncture for curing something that was already improving by natural processes. In other cases, the operative factor is probably a kind of hypnosis, or the placebo effect."

Probably every medical doctor in the world (and every charlatan, too) knows about the placebo effect. You give the patient some colored aspirins or sugar pills, and you tell him he is getting some powerful new miracle drug. It does not work with all patients in all situations, but it works often enough to be a recognized medical phenomenon. The patient feels better because he *believes* he will feel better. You have influenced him with your white coat and other trappings of medical omniscience. The "cure" takes place because of the power of suggestion—what happens in his mind—not because of any properties in the pills or in the acupuncturist's needles.

That was my feeling about acupuncture—a feeling that was shared and is still shared by many Western physicians (and by some in China itself, as a matter of fact).

Some years later, back in America, I began to be troubled by a herniated disk in the lower part of my spine. The pain grew serious, disabling me on some days. I sought all kinds of treatments without getting much relief. For about a year I had to walk around wearing a heavy metal brace. That may have prevented the condition from becoming worse, but it did little to prevent painful spasms.

What could I do? I had to control the pain in some way or I would never get any work done. For complicated reasons, surgery was considered inadvisable. My orthopedic physician recommended what seemed to be an obvious answer: pain-deadening drugs. But when I looked down the long avenue of years ahead of me and saw nothing but rows and rows of pill bottles, I did not like the vision. Would I really be trapped in a life-style of taking drugs to help me struggle through each day?

An opportunity arose for another trip to the East. I was desperate for an answer to my problem, and I decided to try acupuncture. I did not seriously believe it could help, and I feared possible infection from unsterile needles—but I was ready to try almost anything. With the help of a friend and medical colleague in Taipei, and with an English-speaking Chinese nurse as interpreter, I visited a number of acupuncturists in the city's dirty, crowded back streets. I spoke to Chinese patients through my interpreter, and I also spoke to some Americans who had traveled to Taipei for treatments. Many of these men and women claimed amazing results. Some of the results I witnessed were almost as hard to believe.

QUICK HEADACHE RELIEF
WITHOUT DRUGS

I determined to try acupuncture for myself. I remember my first treatment vividly. The acupuncturist practiced in some rooms above a Taipei grocery store. The people in the neighborhood referred to this place as a clinic, but their word did not mean what *clinic* means to a modern American. When you and I hear that word, we think of a place that is brilliantly clean, full of unpleasant but reassuring antiseptic smells. The acupuncture clinic was cluttered and dusty. A strong odor of incense permeated the air. Unscreened windows were open, and flies were buzzing around. I was asked to lie down on a table covered with a soiled sheet and pillowcase. When the acupuncturist began pulling his needles out of a grimy-looking pocket pack, my medical training triumphed over my desire to be polite. I turned to the nurse who had accompanied me and asked her to give him the sterilized needles we had brought with us.

The acupuncturist did not seem offended by this. Undoubtedly he was thinking just about what I was thinking: that East is East and West is West, and the two may never understand each other.

As I lay on the treatment table, my back and leg throbbed painfully. I had unavoidably thrown my back into spasm while walking up the stairs to the clinic. I felt needles prick my skin as the acupuncturist deftly inserted them at several points in my back and shoulders. And then, quite suddenly, I felt no pain at all.

It was hard for me to believe. Yet there it was,

a fact I simply could not deny: The pain in my back
and leg was gone.

In the weeks that followed, I visited that acupuncturist and others, whenever new spasms seized my
back. The treatments always gave me some relief, but
the effects varied greatly according to needle place-
ments. I talked to the practitioners and began to learn
something about their strange art, or science, or whatever it was. One thing I learned was that it is possible
to treat oneself by using the thumbnails or fingernails
in place of a needle. I practiced "finger needle," as the
Chinese call it, and grew adept. In time I was able to
control my pain easily by pressing the indicated body
points whenever a spasm began. I discarded the metal
brace. I no longer needed either the brace or the pain
medicine . . . or the needles, for that matter.

Back home in Illinois, I went on studying acupuncture. I spent thousands of hours trying to work
out a rational explanation of its effects in terms of
Western neurology and neurophysiology. I noted points
of agreement between acupuncture and Western medicine. Where the two seemed to disagree, I tried to
figure out whether the apparent disparity was essential
or real. Or was it mainly a matter of semantics or a result of looking at the same thing from different per-
spectives?

The many-faceted problem of headache had always intrigued and puzzled me. At Evanston Hospital,

---

when dealing with people disabled by life-threatening depressions, we sometimes utilize electroshock therapy. This therapy relieves the symptoms of severe depressions, but it has an unwanted side effect: Immediately after treatment, some patients awaken with agonizing headaches. To deaden the pain, we often gave intramuscular injections of potent narcotics.

As my studies of acupuncture and acupressure progressed, I began to wonder about the possibility of relieving electroshock headaches by thumb pressure instead of drug injections. I worked out a set of pressure points—places on the body where pressure would be expected to relieve a headache if my calculations were correct. I tried the technique on some patients. It worked. In fact, it relieved headaches faster and more surely than narcotic injections.

After using acupressure to alleviate about a hundred post-electroshock headaches, I began using it in my office with outpatients who were suffering from headaches of other kinds. With few exceptions, it worked in those cases, too.

The next step in my long journey, and the most important of all as far as the reader of this book is concerned, came when I taught patients how to use acupressure on themselves. The results? I can only tell you that I converted them, and they confirmed my own conversion of myself, to acupressure as a true breakthrough medical discovery in the relief of suffering from headache pains.

I frequently ask other medical doctors, "Why should anyone take toxic drugs for headache pains when all he has to do to relieve the pains is to press his thumbs in the right ways against the right places?" By the time you have finished reading what I have discovered about acupressure, you will be asking yourself that identical question.

CHAPTER

4

_____

**MEDICAL
SCIENCE
EAST AND
WEST**

THERE ARE TWO things you should know about my approach to medicine: It is empirical and it is eclectic.

Empirical. I observe what works clinically. If something works, I am interested in it. I always ask why and how it works, but I do not necessarily insist on having those questions answered. The questions I do insist on answering are, *Does it work?* and *Is it dangerous?* This empiricism has characterized many aspects of medical science in both East and West. Nobody really knows, for example, how and why aspirin works to deaden pain. There are many theories, but the precise bodily mechanism has not yet been explained to everyone's satisfaction. Despite that gap in our knowledge, we go on using aspirin because we observe that it works. The problem with aspirin and other "pain-killers," of course, is that they produce unwanted and often dangerous side effects, more dangerous than most people realize.

Eclectic. I am willing to study any treatment that impresses me as effective and safe, no matter what school or philosophy of medicine it comes from. I am not a devotee or supporter of any one school. Instead, I prefer to synthesize the best developments of all schools, Eastern or Western, ancient or modern. In my psychiatric practice I use Rorschach inkblot tests sometimes, acupressure sometimes. Each has certain uses and each, when properly applied to those uses, works. To throw away something useful because it is alien to one school or another—to ignore Rorschach because you favor the Orient or acupressure because you favor the West—seems foolish to me.

Conversely, it does not trouble me to discard what seems less useful. It is not necessary to embrace all of Chinese philosophy in order to study or accept acupuncture. Thus you will find little in this book about Yin and Yang and other concepts by which the ancient Oriental practitioners sought to explain their medical observations. It is true that those ancient concepts are fascinating. It is even true that many scientists are investigating the applicability of those ancient concepts to modern medical science. But I have no intention of trying to make that case here. I am interested only in helping you relieve your headache. What is irrelevant to that objective is irrelevant to this book.

Acupuncture, the ancient technique that is the father of acupressure, is not as new a phenomenon in the West as some of today's fad-followers seem to believe. American and European physicians have known about it, studied it, and experimented with it for nearly a century and a half. References to it can be found in American medical journals as far back as the 1830s.

Sir William Osler, a renowned nineteenth-century physician, practiced acupuncture along with Western medical techniques and recommended it for treatment of lumbago and other problems. Osler, sometimes called the father of modern American medicine, was eclectic. He doubted the traditional Oriental teaching that needles must be made of certain metals for certain uses. He found that an ordinary hatpin would serve just as well as an acupuncture needle. And of course he added a Western touch: He insisted that the needles be sterilized.

Acupuncture became an American fad after President Nixon's trip to China in 1972. Journalists and others brought back glowing reports, not always substantiated with factual evidence, on acupuncture's efficacy in curing just about every disease known to man. Dozens of books were published on the topic. Some of the books made sense, some did not, and some were sheer quackery. Simultaneously, thousands of self-styled acupuncturists set up shop in this country and began accepting patients and cash. Few of those practitioners had the necessary training and qualifications. Many had done nothing more than read a couple of those hurriedly published books or attend a weekend seminar.

The acupuncture fad fitted itself neatly into the general Eastward-reaching movement that had already been under way in America since the 1960s. In some circles, the movement doted on Oriental mysticism and, as a corollary, scorned Western pragmatism. The movement had gained a kind of chic currency in many corners of our society by the early 1970s, and few dared suggest in public that some of those mystical teachings might, in fact, be nonsense.

It was all very unfortunate for the serious study of acupuncture. After being introduced into American medical science over a hundred years ago, acupuncture suddenly became associated with a lot of fashionable absurdities. Some wildly exaggerated claims were made for it—and the more absurd the claim, the more readily some people seemed to accept it.

One often-repeated claim, for example, was that acupuncture can be used to produce anesthesia for surgical operations. An article in a mystical cultists' publication went so far as to say that this "acuthesia" wafts you into an ecstatic, otherworldly state in which your consciousness somehow leaves your body, and you watch the operation as though from a seat in the clouds. This was perfect nonsense. Acupuncture cannot and does not produce surgical anesthesia. What it can produce, when properly applied, is analgesia—or, to put it more precisely, hypalgesia, the *lessening* of pain sensations.

All this Eastern-mystical ballyhoo hampered American physicians who were seriously trying to find where and how acupuncture might be welcomed into modern Western medical science. Partly at their urging, various federal and state government agencies have recently turned their attention to acupuncture and have sought to find what its advantages and disadvantages really are. The National Institutes of Health and other federal agencies have sponsored studies and conferences on the subject. The California Board of Medical Examiners and the New York State Board for Medicine have also been prominent in this effort to get at the truth in a cool, rational way.

The results are beginning to show, and they are good. The circus atmosphere is slowly diminishing, giving way to honest scientific inquiry. Most state medical boards and other groups that have studied acupuncture have now recommended that it be accorded the same respect—and also subjected to the same regulations—as any other medical procedure that is demonstrably useful but on which research still needs to be done.

But the harm done in those circus years following 1972 has not been wiped away—not by any means. The

QUICK HEADACHE RELIEF
WITHOUT DRUGS

New York State Commission on Acupuncture interviewed physicians who were skeptical about the technique and tried to find out why. Many of those skeptical doctors, it turned out, were unhappy about the "commercial exploitation and charlatanism" that were so prevalent at the height of the fad. Others were turned off by "the ancient and obsolete philosophical explanations of Yin and Yang," and other mystical trappings with which acupuncture had been festooned.

There is still a lot of skepticism in the air. If there is any of it in you, I must obviously overcome it before I can persuade you to put any faith in auto-acupressure.

How and why does acupuncture, and hence acupressure, work? As the New York State Commission on Acupuncture put it, that is "still a mystery after five thousand years."

Not wholly a mystery, perhaps. A widely accepted view, which my own research leads me to agree with, is that the effects work somehow through the peripheral, autonomic and central nervous systems. Many of the main acupuncture points, including those that apply to headaches, are located along nerve pathways with which any Western neurologist is familiar. What is not clearly understood (as with aspirin) is the exact neural mechanism that produces the effects.

The science of acupuncture probably began with

simple, empirical observations. Ancient Oriental doctors or philosophers, thousands of years ago, may have
noticed that something going wrong in one part of the
body can produce pain in another part. Angina pectoris,
a heart condition, is a dramatic example. The pain is
felt not only in the chest but also, commonly, in the
left arm. We call this "referred pain." An example that
may be more familiar to you is toothache. The pain can
spread through your whole jaw, even throughout your
head. It may become so diffuse that you cannot determine which tooth is actually causing the problem.
When I begin teaching you auto-acupressure, I will
show you other examples of referred pain that may surprise you. For instance, when you have a headache
there are points on your body, often far removed from
the head, that grow perceptibly tender to any pressure
applied.

This observation of referred pain may have given
those ancient Oriental practitioners some ideas for treatment. One of their major problems must have been
that they could not examine organs inside the body,
as we can today. They were even limited in their
ability to perform ordinary physical examinations, the
kind most modern Americans take for granted. Women
would not undress for such an examination. Instead of
looking at his patient's body, the ancient Chinese physician often had to make "diagnoses" with a small doll

of a reclining woman. The patient would indicate what and where her own complaints were by pointing to various parts of the doll.

Laws and social customs in ancient China also discouraged anatomical studies of the deceased, which, again, Western medical scientists and students have long taken for granted. Since they could not examine the inside of the body, those ancient Orientals were attracted to the idea that problems inside might be treated by manipulating areas on the outside.

Gradually, by trial and error, by seeing what worked and what did not, they arrived at systems of treatment that seemed useful. Needling was not the only such system. There were treatment methods, for example, in which stones were rubbed on the body. But acupuncture has survived the best, presumably because it worked the best.

As the centuries went by, acupuncture systems became more refined and more elaborate. We know of many such systems today, originating from various countries and regions of the East. In most of the systems, between five hundred and eight hundred body points or loci are associated with various organs and various diseases. The systems differ in detail, but the differences are less striking than the similarities. All the systems, of course, depend on external manipulation. And in most of them, the more important loci are in the same places.

Having developed an empirical system that worked, the ancient Chinese did what any thinking person would do: They sought to explain why it worked. The idea that a needle placed outside the body could produce effects inside must have been as puzzling to them as it was, later, to Western observers. In an attempt to make sense of the phenomenon, they built an elaborate philosophical structure around it. They envisioned a universal life-energy force called Ch'i, which flows through the body under the control of negative and positive forces called Yin and Yang. In their analysis, sickness resulted when Yin and Yang slipped out of balance in various parts of the body and in various ways, and normal, healthy balance was restored by placing needles in the appropriate spots.

This explanation (which I have vastly oversimplified for the sake of brevity) satisfied the ancient Chinese. If it does not satisfy us today, we need not throw acupuncture out with it. The ancients in our own half of the world believed thunder and lightning were caused by angry gods. We do not believe that explanation today, but we have not therefore decided to stop believing in thunder and lightning. They plainly exist. We see and hear them with our own eyes and ears, and we are at liberty to favor any other explanation that makes more sense to us.

So it is with acupuncture. And with the subject of this book—acupressure. It demonstrably works, as your headaches, or, rather, your relief from the pain they cause, will tell you by the time you finish this book. The effects plainly exist. We can use those effects without needing to accept a distant culture's explanation of *why* they exist.

Modern Chinese medicine shows an eclecticism very much like mine. Those journalists who accompanied President Nixon were perfectly correct in saying acupuncture is used today in Chinese hospitals. What the reporters did not always stress was that it is often used together with modern Western techniques.

Western ideas dominated Chinese medicine earlier in this century. There was a long period when acupuncture was officially frowned upon. Among intellectuals and most city dwellers who thought of themselves as "modern," it was pretty well discredited as mere old-time superstition. It survived mainly in the rural area, where it was practiced by paramedical practitioners generally called "barefoot doctors."

Late in the 1940s, under Chairman Mao, acupuncture and other traditional approaches were lifted out of this limbo of official scorn. Mao's thought was, "Let's keep what works." Western-trained Chinese physicians began working side by side with traditional acupuncturists and herb doctors. The result is a mixed breed of medical science: part East, part West.

Acupuncture is used to produce hypalgesia in some surgical operations, for instance, but it is often used in conjunction with local anesthetics, tranquilizers, and analgesics.

American medicine has progressed by incorporating discoveries from all over the world and from many centuries. Many modern medicines, for instance, have been derived from roots, barks, and plants used in treatment since antiquity. There is no reason why acupressure (and its parent, acupuncture) can't be welcomed and utilized for the benefit of mankind in the same way.

CHAPTER

5

YOUR
HEADACHE
OR
YOUR LIFE

You MAY WONDER at this point why I do not get down to the cure instead of continuing to talk about the symptoms. As a trained physician and practicing specialist I am particularly aware of the need for careful medical diagnosis. Until I have given you the reasons why, as far as we know them, you cannot fully understand the methods how. What I have to say in this chapter is important background information for everyone who suffers from headaches and, especially, from migraine and tension headaches.

It is estimated that more than ninety percent of American adults and teen-agers occasionally get headaches that are severe and long-lasting enough to interfere with pleasure and lower efficiency in work and play. (Children get headaches, too, and there is evidence that even babies do, but there is no agreement on the number or severity.)

Another estimate is that forty to fifty million Americans—perhaps a quarter of the population—at various times have headaches that are painful enough to cause definite disruptions of their lives. These are the head-aches that make people change plans, stop work, stay home from their jobs and schools, miss leisure-time events, and leave parties early. Of those forty to fifty million people, the estimate is that close to half find themselves in so much pain, at one time or another, that they must go to bed for a while.

These fifty million headaches are of many different kinds, with many different causes. Some signify nothing much more than that your head hurts; that is, the head-pain symptom itself is the worst part of the disease. These are by far the most common types of headaches, and they are the types you can treat effectively with auto-acupressure. Other kinds, much less common, signify that something is seriously wrong somewhere in the body, and in these cases it is perilous to treat the head-pain symptom alone.

In this chapter and the next, I want to tell you something of what, in my extensive work as a neurologist and as a psychiatrist, I have learned about headaches. The more fully you understand that ache in your head, the more efficiently and safely you will be able to banish it. In headache treatment, as in poker, business, and war, it is hazardous to assault an opponent you have not reconnoitered.

Let us start by looking at four case histories from my files: the stories of two men and two women. Each of them suffered from a common type of headache. I have chosen these four cases because they illustrate that headaches, though superficially alike, can spring from quite different bodily and emotional mechanisms.

Lost Weekends: I. George R. was a big, florid-faced man in his middle thirties, friendly, outgoing, cheerful. In high school and college he had played football, but his once-athletic body was now beginning to show the results of too much good eating and too little exercise. He played golf once in a while but it did not help much. He was overweight and starting to develop a paunch.

He had a highly paid, responsible job as an assistant sales chief in a company that manufactured industrial chemicals. He had started working for this company as a young on-the-road salesman. By putting in 'long hours and paying close attention to political structures within the company, he had broken sales records, established himself early as a bright young climber, and gained the attention of the company's top executives. In promoting him through divisional levels and finally to his present job, they had moved him up much faster than people in that company normally moved. The job he now held had never before been filled by any man under forty.

George liked his work. He found it exciting and

challenging. It required him to travel a lot and often work far into the night, but this did not trouble him greatly. "If you want a nine-to-five job, then you've got to be happy with nine-to-five pay," he said, summing up his philosophy. "Me, I'm willing to work harder for more. Frankly, I like money and I want all I can get. And it isn't as though I find the work a big burden. My job gives me a lot of satisfaction, and I'm good at it and I don't mind putting a lot of effort into it."

George's salary, plus profit-sharing bonuses, enabled him to afford a big, sumptuous house with a swimming pool in a fashionable high-income community. He had a wife and three children. His only regret about his job was that it prevented him from seeing his family as often as he wished.

He had experienced headaches occasionally in high school and college. He recalled that they often came on after a football game. "I'd be taking a shower after the game, or maybe getting ready to go out with a girl that night, and *wham!* it would hit me, a headache that knocked the wind out of me. It would come on hard, but I'd take a couple of aspirins and I'd be OK after a while. The next morning I'd be fine. In those days, I never had a headache that lasted more than a few hours."

After college and until about age thirty, he was fairly free of headaches. "Once in a while I'd drink too much and wake up with a hangover headache," he recalled. "And sometimes I'd get what I guess you'd call a 'hunger' headache. It was usually after one of those superbusy days at work, you know? The kind of day when you skip meals, try to get by on snacks and coffee. At night I'd have a dull headache, nothing very bad. Except for that, I was pretty much headache-free through most of my twenties."

One Friday night, shortly after his thirtieth birthday, he was riding homeward on a plane from a distant city, where he had attended a sales meeting. As he sipped his second Scotch-on-the-rocks, he began to notice a dull, throbbing pain in the left side of his head, behind the eye. He finished his drink. The pain grew worse. He asked the stewardess for two aspirins. The aspirins did not help. The pain was still there when he got off the plane, and it was growing worse.

By the time he arrived home, he was in anguish. He went to bed with two more aspirins, slept badly, awoke the next morning with the headache somewhat abated but still decidedly there. It stayed with him all weekend, more bearable at some hours than others, but never quite gone. And then, when he awoke on Monday morning, he felt better. By midmorning, there was no more pain.

A few weekends later, the headache came back. The onset was as before: a throbbing pain behind the left eye. It arrived this time on a Saturday morning, just as he was preparing to take one of his sons to a Little League baseball game. He made it to the game, but the pain grew to such severity that he had to leave early. As he drove home, the agony became so intense that he squinted his left eye shut and clutched that side of his head with his hand. "I was driving one-eyed and one-handed. It's lucky I didn't smash up my car. The pain was horrible, like a red-hot poker being plunged in and out the left side of my skull."

At home, he lay down on a sofa. His wife went out to buy an "extrastrength pain reliever" at the local drugstore. The pills deadened the pain somewhat, but new symptoms appeared as the day wore on. George found himself sweating profusely. His vision was blurred, and he felt nauseated. He ate virtually nothing that day, slept fitfully, awoke early on Sunday morning with the same intense agony behind his left eye. Worse, the pain now seemed to have spread to the other side of his head. "It seemed to go all the way through my head and back to the hinge of my jaw. Even my teeth hurt."

On Monday, as before, the headache went away.

And so it went, every second or third weekend. George came to dread weekends. He was afraid to make plans for Saturday and Sunday because he never knew when those plans would have to be called off.

His wife faced the same difficulty. She had to keep backing out of social engagements with the excuse, "George has one of his headaches." She came to hate the sound of the words. She wondered if friends always believed she was speaking the truth.

A headache is perfectly real to the sufferer, but it may not always look real to other people. There are no visible symptoms—at least, none that are readily visible to the untrained eye. Everybody knows that a faked headache can be used to back out of anything you do not want to do, be it work or play. The faked headache has probably been used as an excuse since the dawn of polite society. George's wife was embarrassed and unhappy. She had greatly enjoyed their weekends together. Now their friends were cooling off on them, and she was stuck at home with a man who was irritable and preoccupied with his pains and aches.

It was at his wife's urging that George came to see me. Her theory was that his headaches were of purely psychogenic origin. This is a popular diagnosis, often heard, not so often true. "It's all in your head," people tell the headache sufferer. They think he is "imagining" it, or they postulate that he has some obscure emotional problem that has somehow been translated into a false sensation of pain in the head.

It turned out that George's headaches were indeed triggered by emotional events. But to say that there was no tangible physical cause for all that pain would have been grossly inaccurate. His pain was as real as the pain from a cut finger or a bruised shin.

I gave him a thorough neurological examination. Except for his overweight condition and a few other more minor problems, he was in good health. I told him that, and then I told him why his head hurt on weekends. He was a victim of letdown migraine.

The word *migraine* is derived from Greek roots meaning "half head." This kind of headache often (though not always) attacks one side of the head, or starts on one side. The direct physical cause is dilation of arteries within the skull. When these blood vessels expand, they pull on nerves surrounding them. This traction on the nerves is what causes the peculiarly agonizing effects of migraine.

What is the cause behind the cause? What makes the arteries dilate? There are, unfortunately, many possibilities. The effects can be brought on by allergies, for example, allergies to pollens or other airborne substances, or to foods. Or the dilation of blood vessels might occur because of an imbalance in the nervous system, perhaps resulting from emotional factors. The sufferer might have a tendency to react allergically to certain foods, for instance, but might experience no difficulty from this under normal circumstances. The allergic symptoms might show up, however, when his or her bodily defenses are weakened by emotional stress. Result: migraine headaches in periods of hectic work or family strife.

The "letdown migraine," which comes on *after* a period of stress, is fairly common. This was George's problem. Whenever he was letting down and trying to relax after a hard-driving week, changes took place in his nervous system. On weekends when the changes were pronounced enough, blood vessels in his head dilated and he was incapacitated.

We'll get back to George later. Now for Clare.

Lost Weekends: II. Clare N. was a small, soft-voiced woman in her early thirties. She had long dark hair and an appealing air of shyness. She had led a sheltered childhood in a small, sleepy southern town, where she was surrounded by a large, loving, protective family. She was the youngest of seven brothers and sisters, the adored and pampered baby of the family. In other homes nearby lived grandparents, uncles, aunts, cousins. It was a cozy world for a girl to grow up in, but it was not a world that prepared her well for life beyond its borders. Nobody demanded much of Clare, and she had little practice in self-assertiveness or in trying to find solutions to her own problems. If something or somebody troubled her, she ran to a parent or an older brother or an aunt, and everything was made right.

At age eighteen she went away to college. The

campus seemed to her a cold, unfeeling place, full of aggressive people who were pursuing their own dreams and purposes and had neither the time nor the inclination to pay attention to her. Lonely, homesick, a little scared, she dropped out and fled back to the shelter of her family.

During those months at college, she experienced her first cluster headaches. They often began in her sleep. She would awaken with a grinding pain in the region of one temple or the other, sometimes both. The agony was so intense that it brought tears to her eyes. The pain might last for five or ten minutes, then subside. Sometimes a new attack would begin minutes later. At other times several hours might go by with no new attack. She would assume the cluster was ended, only to feel a sudden new spear of pain while walking to class or sitting in the library. On several occasions she had to run from a classroom or lecture hall with tears running down her cheeks. These embarrassing episodes made her all the more shy. She was sure her classmates thought her odd.

Back home in the bosom of her family, she talked about her headaches with an older cousin, a nurse. The nurse offered the opinion that the headaches were "only tension" and prescribed tranquillity and aspirin. Clare had already prescribed aspirin for herself but had not found it very helpful. She did notice, however,

---

that the clusters came less and less frequently in the calm atmosphere of her home environment.

After dropping out of college and a year of living at home, working as a secretary in a local bank, she found that her headaches were virtually gone. They forced her to stay at home from work three or four days a year at the most.

Carl, a former high school friend of Clare's, returned to town after graduating from college one summer. He and Clare saw each other often, and at the end of the summer he asked her to marry him. Life in her parents' home had been tranquil, but also boring. She said yes.

Carl was an executive trainee in a large corporation with plants and offices all over the country. As he was promoted up the income levels, he and Clare moved from city to city. When he worked his way up to a responsible job in the corporation's Chicago headquarters, they bought a large suburban home and settled there with their two children.

Clare's headache clusters now began to be a problem again. For several years they had been infrequent, usually mild and of short duration. Now they came once a month or so and lasted a day, two days, sometimes three. What puzzled Clare and upset Carl was that they often occurred on weekends.

Carl's executive job—or, to state the case more accurately, his own ambitions in the job—required him to do a lot of entertaining: colleagues, customers, visiting associates from other cities. It was his theory that a lot of good business could be done and much good will gained when men and wives met for cocktails, dinners, and evenings at the theater. Beyond that, he was a gregarious man, as well as one with a consuming interest in social status. He wanted to rank high in the social environment of their suburban community. He and Clare had joined a country club, and their social life was an active one.

More active, in fact, than Clare wanted it to be. She liked some of the people she met but found many of them "too loud and pushy," as she put it. She had never been an assertive woman, and she felt lost in this world of aggressive, overwhelmingly self-assured people. "I feel as though they're all waiting for me to make a mistake," she sometimes said. What kind of mistake? She didn't know, but the feeling was there nonetheless.

She was particularly unhappy when she had to be Carl's hostess at a business-oriented dinner or cocktail party. "I hate having to smile at a lot of people I don't really like," she told Carl one night after a theater outing. He reacted with anger. "We're supposed to be partners!" he shouted. "If you like living in a nice home and driving a new car, you've got to help me earn the money that makes those things possible."

One Friday afternoon, as Clare was preparing canapés for a party the following night, she began to notice some strange sensations. There was a peculiar feeling around her temples. It was very hard to describe, but she said later that it felt as though the skin there was alternately wrinkling and stretching, "the way an accordion does." There were also bright spots floating in front of her eyes. They looked something like slowly drifting dust motes seen in a ray of bright sunshine.

These odd effects were to become depressingly familiar to her in years to come. She was experiencing the aura that sometimes comes before headaches of a certain type. Not every attack is preceded by such an aura, but when it does turn up, it is an all too reliable warning signal. Headaches follow inexorably.

The headache cluster that attacked her that night, and remained throughout the weekend, was excruciating. There were other symptoms in addition to the pain. Her nose was runny, as though she had a cold. Her eyes were red and watery, and her face swelled.

The party had to be called off. Carl tried to be sympathetic but did not do a good job of it. By the end of the weekend his anger was showing.

((81))

QUICK HEADACHE RELIEF
WITHOUT DRUGS

Weekend after weekend, the same unhappy drama was played out. Clare's condition grew worse. Finally, she was unable to do any entertaining at all. It was rare that she was even able to go to any weekend social event without getting struck down by a headache.

Clare tried drugs, folk remedies, everything she could think of. Aspirin, Dristan, Excedrin, and other over-the-counter drugs took the edge off the pain, but they upset her stomach when she took them continuously for more than a day. She played the frustrating game of "maybe I'm allergic to this or that." Allergic to what? Well, perhaps to alcohol. She had never been much of a drinker, but now she tried drinking only plain fruit juice or ginger ale at parties. That didn't help. She read a magazine article about people who are allergic to dairy products, and she swore off butter, eggs, and milk. Nothing changed. Carl suggested that she give up tea, which she loved. She tried that, with no results. Learning from a friend that carbon monoxide can cause headaches, she kept her car windows open even in freezing weather. This did nothing but make her cold.

Carl grew impatient, angry, sarcastic. "We might as well rent a cave and become hermits," he said one Saturday as she lay miserably in bed. "I can't go on living like this, Clare. I work hard all week, and then on weekends I want to have some fun. What kind of life is this? I'm not married to a wife anymore. I'm married to a headache."

When Clare came to see me, I examined her carefully. The examination confirmed a guess I could have given when she first told me about her symptoms. They were the classic symptoms of *histamine cephalgia*, or the "cluster" headache.

Histamine is a chemical produced by various body cells. When emotional upset or some other triggering event occurs in men and women who are predisposed to this problem, something goes wrong with the body's control system, and too much histamine is released. It can cause, among other things, dilation of blood vessels, congestion in the nose and sinuses, watering of the eyes, and a red blotchy swollen appearance in the face. For reasons that are too complicated to sort out here (and that are not perfectly understood in any case), histamine headaches almost always have that peculiar "clustering" characteristic. There is a sharp pain, usually in the temple region or behind the eye, followed by a pain-free or nearly pain-free period, followed by more pain.

Since these headaches are caused by dilation of arteries in the head, they are loosely classified as a type of migraine. The pain of histamine cephalgia is often more intense, however, than that of common migraine headaches. Because of this, and because of the off-and-on characteristic of this kind of headache, its victims sometimes take enormous amounts of drugs. The sufferer is never quite sure when a cluster has ended. Fearing new pain spasms, he or she may go on taking pain-relieving drugs for days after a cluster has subsided.

Lost Weekends: III. Clare's husband, Carl, had headaches too, but of an entirely different kind from his wife's. The pain generally began at the back of his head and neck, then spread forward over his scalp. During the most severe attacks, he felt as though the entire top of his head was being squeezed in a vise.

As his weekend arguments with Clare increased in frequency and severity, so did his headaches. In the past Carl's headaches had occurred in a seemingly random pattern, perhaps one every two or three months, but now they began to occur more and more often on weekends. The more severe they became, the less patient he was with his wife. He began to think of her as a burden—and when he had a headache, he bluntly told her so. Sometimes, when they both had headaches they would spend an entire weekend in sullen silence, broken only by an occasional bitter argument in which both of them blurted out hurtful and regrettable words. They began to avoid each other, slept in separate beds, even ate meals separately.

They seemed to be trapped in a self-feeding spiral of head pain and emotional misery. Carl was a victim of *muscle-contraction headaches,* often, not quite accurately, called "tension" headaches. The pain was caused by hours long or days long tightness of muscles in his neck, scalp, and face. This tightness was brought on by the frustrations and anger in him—unhappy feelings that, in turn, were brought on at least partly by Clare's headaches.

A muscle-contraction headache can sometimes be eliminated by taking time away from the stressful situation that is causing it, or by sheer physical exertion—playing tennis, for instance, or scrubbing a floor. It might help to have an emotional escape, such as reading an absorbing book, or simply by getting a good night's sleep. But it is not always possible to escape from a stressful situation. This was Carl's problem. Headaches seemed to be driving him and Clare toward a divorce. We will have more to say about Clare and Carl, but first let us look at the problem of Annette.

Lost Weekends: IV. Annette J. was a single woman in her middle twenties. She consulted me because, for about two years, she had found herself awakening with headaches on Saturday mornings. The headaches were sometimes so painful that she had to spend much of the day in bed and cancel Saturday-

---

night plans. I gave her the usual examination and found her in excellent health. My initial guess was that she might be suffering from letdown migraine like George R., but it was a guess that turned out to be wrong.

Annette told me about her life. She had been born into a family that never had quite enough money. Throughout her early life in a dreary Pennsylvania mill town, she had read avidly of glamorous worlds far away and had resolved to leave her hometown far behind. "There were two things I dreamed of when I was in high school," she said. "One was life in a big city, and the other was travel. I wanted to see Europe, the Orient—all those far-off places I read about in magazines."

She worked hard in school and won a scholarship to a nearby college. She came out with a degree in economics, landed a fairly high-paying job in the economic-research department of a major bank, and finally realized her dream of living in an apartment of her own in a big city. She saved her money carefully, and each summer she and some friends took a two-week vacation in some exotic land across the sea.

She seemed to me an unusually contented, happy woman. She had achieved some major childhood dreams at an early age. She enjoyed her work at the bank. Her job and her attitude toward it seemed to lack the pressures that drove George R. to a state of near-exhaustion each Friday. "I work hard," she told me, "but the atmosphere is relaxed and friendly. It's a job where I can more or less make my own schedule. It isn't a rat race. I wouldn't want a job if it made me too tired to enjoy my evenings."

She had found many friends in the big city. One group of single men and women made a point of meeting each Friday night at a restaurant not far from the bank. They customarily had a few drinks, ate dinner, talked far into the night about their ambitions, the state of the world, the traveling they wanted to do. "It's almost like a club," she said. "Sometimes we make plans to go to a museum or something on Saturday—but of course with these headaches I've been getting lately, I often have to beg off."

I asked her what she drank at these Friday-night gatherings. Alcohol is a poison, though most adults can drink moderate amounts without severe effects. Like any other poison—carbon monoxide, for example, is another common one—it can cause headache if the body takes in more than it can tolerate at one time. But Annette told me she usually drank only a glass or two of wine. "I sometimes drink that much on other nights of the week," she said. "But I hardly ever get a headache after those other nights—only on Saturday."

She went on to tell me she had heard about my

auto-acupressure technique from a friend and was eager to try it. "I'm fascinated by the East," she said, smiling. "I've been there twice, and I'm thinking about Hong Kong this summer. I've got Oriental rugs in my apartment, Chinese paintings, Chinese vases. . . . So you can see why anything like acupressure would interest me."

A thought suddenly occurred to me. "This place where your group meets on Friday nights," I said. "What kind of restaurant is it?"

She laughed. "I'll give you one guess. It's a Chinese restaurant, of course."

"Do you eat Chinese food on other nights of the week?"

"No, almost never. Most nights I cook myself a lamb chop or a hamburger, whatever is on sale at the supermarket."

I nodded. "I'd like you to try something," I said. "For the next few Friday nights, see if you can get your friends to meet somewhere else—any other kind of restaurant just as long as it isn't Chinese. Maybe your headaches will vanish."

The clues she had given me made me suspect what is sometimes called CRS, the "Chinese restaurant syndrome." Chinese cooking employs a large amount of monosodium glutamate—a flavor enhancer—and there is also a high concentration of it in soy sauce. Many people react allergically to this chemical. The chief symptom is usually an agonizing headache.

Annette phoned me a few weeks later to tell me my diagnosis had been correct. She had talked the group into changing their meeting place. They now met in an Italian restaurant. Ever since the change had been made, she had awakened on Saturdays headache-free.

These four cases illustrate four common kinds of headaches. Of the four, only Annette's could be treated by simply removing the cause. The other three sufferers—George, Clare, and her husband, Carl—had headaches of more complicated origin, and in their cases the only practical approach was to treat the pain with auto-acupressure. I am happy to say that all three now have their headaches comfortably under control. Exactly how I treated them—and taught them to treat themselves—will be described in detail in the subsequent chapters.

I have presented the four cases in this way because it is hard to talk about a headache without also talking about the person who has it. Obviously a headache never exists in the abstract. It is always in somebody's head.

This is why nearly all attempts to label headaches as types and subtypes have run into difficulty. No matter how carefully you draw up your classifications, there will always be many headaches that do not fit those classifications well. You might identify a Type A headache, for instance, or a Type B, C, or D. But only sometimes will you meet someone who has a perfect Type A headache as you have described and classified it. More often, you will have to be content to say, "Well, yes, this person has a *kind* of Type A headache, but with elements of Type B and maybe a touch of Type C."

One classification system, for instance, makes a distinction between "associative" headaches and "chronic" ones. A chronic headache might be a migraine or muscle-contraction headache, one that recurs frequently and in the same way over some appreciable span of time. An associative headache, in this classification, would be one that is associated with a one-time event such as a fever, or an occasional event such as alcohol hangover, or a seasonal event such as a spring-pollen allergy. But this classification leads to confusion. A migraine sufferer might be subject to all three of those associative influences I have just named, and more. In that particular sufferer, the nervous-system imbalance that brings on migraine symptoms might result from fever, drinking too much, spring pollen, and perhaps a dozen other factors. What should his or her headaches be called? Chronic or associative?

There have also been attempts to distinguish between "organically caused" and "emotionally caused" headaches. There are, indeed, headaches that point to serious organic disorders. But the most common headaches are hard to classify in this way. As the stories of George R. and Clare N. show pretty clearly, both physical and emotional factors may be involved in a given headache attack—involved in such a way that it is impossible to separate the two. Carl's muscle-contraction headaches were perhaps more clearly "emotional" in origin; but in his case, too, there was a tangible and perfectly real physical cause for his pain. The pain came from chronically taut muscles. Only Annette's headaches could be classified as clearly organic; but even in her case, it is possible that unknown emotional factors made her body less resistant to the monosodium glutamate reaction on some Saturdays than on others.

As far as auto-acupressure is concerned, there is no need to make fine distinctions among various types of headaches. But if you suffer from headaches, whether occasionally or frequently, it would be negligent of me, as a physician, not to give you the benefit of my experience and sketch in the background information for you. I want you to understand the origins of your headaches as clearly as you can—and I emphatically want you to make sure, by consulting a medical doctor, that no serious physical problem is lurking in the background. However, it won't be necessary for you to classify your pain as "Type B, Subtype 6." In this book, for purposes of teaching you auto-acupressure, I will divide headaches into three broadly defined groups.

Group One. This is the largest group. It includes almost all the common headaches in which no serious medical problems are involved. In this group are migraine and histamine cephalgia (often called "vascular" headaches because they involve blood vessels in the head), and also muscle-contraction or tension headaches.

All these varieties of pain are treated substantially alike in auto-acupressure. No matter where your headache comes from or what it feels like, if it is in this group, you treat it by pressing the same body points in the same ways. If there is no serious underlying physical problem, I can safely and effectively recommend auto-acupressure as the primary treatment for pain of this kind.

Group Two. A smaller group: sinus headaches. There are two reasons for treating sinus headaches as a separate category. One is that you will treat them differently in auto-acupressure; the pressure points are not the same as those of Group One. Another reason for considering sinus headaches separately is that they can sometimes point to a dangerous infection. I do not want you to treat them casually, and I am going to emphasize the potential danger later in this book by putting these headaches in a category by themselves. But remember that, although this type of headache may have an underlying cause that requires medical attention, the painful symptoms can still be relieved by auto-acupressure.

Group Three. The smallest group: headaches that are symptoms of serious disease or damage. These are headaches that you should *not* treat with auto-acupressure, unless your doctor specifically allows you to do so while he treats the underlying cause. We will look at these Group Three headaches in the next chapter.

The common headaches of Group One have long been a source of frustration in Western medical science. One problem is that there are so many possible causes for such headaches. Another problem is that, in light of the fact that these headaches reflect no dangerous illness, it would be too difficult or too expensive to isolate people from the causes. The cure, in other words, would be more trouble than the disease.

For example, a physician might determine that your migraines are caused partly by an airborne allergen of some kind—perhaps a chemical irritant in industrial fumes, perhaps mold spores or something else of natural origin. But what good does this knowledge do you or him? Except in a matter of life or death, he cannot isolate you from the air around you.

Or he might determine that your headaches are caused in whole or in part by emotional stress or its aftereffect, as in the case of George R., the man with letdown migraine. But it is hard to isolate such a man from the stresses in his life. Not even a long and costly course of psychotherapy could be guaranteed to make him immune to that stress—even if George agreed to spend the money and time. Stress is a part of human life. Its effects can be alleviated but hardly ever removed.

George, you will recall, liked his work and willingly put hard effort into it. The obvious and banal pieces of advice—relax, slow down, don't work so hard —would go in one of George's ears and out the other. He was a man who had designed his life in a way that brought him satisfaction. Even though his headaches were painful and he wanted very much to get rid of them, it would be unrealistic to expect that he would revise his life-style for that purpose. Some headache sufferers have found their agony so intolerable that they have been forced to change their life-styles, but this is a drastic measure, a last resort.

Only rarely does it turn out that the cause of a

---

headache can be removed without great trouble and expense. The story of Annette J. is one of those rare, happy cases.

In another case, a woman complained of headaches when reading. She could read for about an hour without discomfort, but after two hours she would find a headache building up around the top of her head, and if she read for much longer than that, the pain grew massive. Since she was a magazine editor, this was more than a trivial problem to her.

She theorized that these were "eyestrain" headaches. This was, in fact, unlikely. Eye injuries and certain eye diseases can cause or contribute to headaches, but there is no evidence that simply *using* the eyes can produce head pain by itself. Most so-called eyestrain headaches are actually muscle-contraction headaches. In any case, there was nothing seriously wrong with the woman's eyes. She went to an ophthalmologist to have her eyes and reading glasses checked, and he found everything in order. She did not need new glasses, he said. On the basis of his examination, there was no reason why reading should cause any discomfort.

The magazine editor might have gone away baffled except for the lucky fact that she asked for the ophthalmologist's bill before she left. As she leaned over a table in his waiting room, writing out her check, he noticed something.

((95))

"Let me see those glasses," he said.

It turned out that the earpieces were loose. The doctor had noticed that the glasses began to slip down her nose as she wrote her check. To keep them from slipping farther, she made an awkward facial grimace and also tensed her scalp so as to pull her ears back. An hour or more of this tension would very easily bring on a headache.

She had the earpieces adjusted so that they clung to her head more securely. The headaches vanished.

Unfortunately, it is rare that a headache story can be brought to so quick, tidy, and satisfying an end. In the vast majority of cases, the causes of headaches are complicated and hard to approach in a practical way.

There has been a good deal of headache research in America during the past few decades, and as a result we now know much more about headache mechanisms than physicians did in 1950. But in many instances, the new knowledge has served only to increase the frustrations. Only occasionally has a newly discovered fact led to a new, simple, inexpensive treatment. Most often, new knowledge has done little more than make the practical problems of Group One headaches seem more complex and baffling.

For instance, there is evidence that a tendency toward migraine headaches is to some extent inheritable. If you are a migraine sufferer and have a friend who is not, the statistical odds are that there will be more migraine sufferers in past and present generations of your family than in your friend's. This interesting piece of knowledge may someday contribute to the discovery of a practical treatment or prevention method, but so far it has not.

Similarly, some researchers believe that headaches may sometimes be precipitated by hormonal changes in the body. In a surprisingly large number of cases, women who suffer from migraine find they have fewer and milder headaches when they are pregnant than when they are not. Sometimes the headaches go away entirely, only to return soon after the baby is born or after lactation stops. Some women find that they are more likely to get headaches when menstruating than at other times of the month, and some find their headaches diminished or virtually gone after menopause. Still other women have found their migraines more frequent and more severe in periods when they were taking birth-control pills. (Many physicians feel that the increase in migraine headaches caused by birth-control pills mandates stopping the pills. There is a statistically significant association between oral contraceptives and cerebral thrombosis.) But again, these observations have not led to a safe, practical new treatment for common migraine.

Observations of and theories about the so-called

headache personality have similarly failed to do much for Group One sufferers. Many writers on the topic have claimed that the typical migraine victim is ambitious, hard-driving, competitive, and a perfectionist; that he or she tends to talk fast and in a loud, high voice, and so on. Victims of muscle-contraction headaches are said to be much the same. In support of this observation, the writers marshal an impressive lineup of famous headache sufferers who allegedly fit the description. Among those most often mentioned are Charles Darwin, Virginia Woolf, Lewis Carroll (who is said to have written parts of *Alice's Adventures in Wonderland* while hallucinating during a migraine attack), President Ulysses S. Grant, and Edgar Allen Poe (whose headaches were so agonizing that he sometimes rushed outdoors to bury his head in snow).

Even if these observations were trustworthy, they would not be of much use in helping you ease the pain in *your* head. They are not very trustworthy in any case. It is true that many people whose heads hurt are ambitious, competitive, loud-voiced, and all that. But there are also many ambitious, competitive, loud-voiced people whose heads do not hurt. And there are many victims of both migraine and muscle-contraction headaches who are not notably ambitious, who are slow-moving and outwardly tranquil, and who talk in soft voices.

And so the common headache, like the common cold, has remained a puzzle and a challenge to Western medical science. Before a therapy for this kind of headache can be considered really useful, it must meet four criteria: It must be effective, safe, practical, and affordable. The search for such a therapy has led researchers down many pathways, but nearly every preventive or treatment method so far developed has failed at least one of those four tests.

There has been a good deal of interest in recent years, for example, in a technique called "biofeedback." It is used for many purposes, including headache treatment. The essential idea of it is to help patients control certain body functions that are not normally thought of as being voluntarily controllable. In the case of hypertension or high blood pressure, for instance, the patient is connected to a monitoring device that measures his blood pressure constantly and shows its readings on a dial. He is asked to watch the dial and try to make his pressure drop. After a good deal of practice, some patients are reportedly able to do it.

There have been several attempts to treat headaches with this technique. One approach began with the observation that people afflicted with severe migraine tend to have cold hands. Simply warming the hands before a fire produces no results, so the researchers turned to biofeedback. Their theory was that, if a patient could warm his own hands by some inner effort of will, he might simultaneously produce other bodily changes that would alleviate his headaches. With at least some patients, the technique appeared to work. But not all test subjects could produce the desired hand-warming effect at will; and of those who could, not all reported significant improvement in their headache problems.

In any case, the main trouble with biofeedback techniques is that, for most people, they are not practical. To become adept at controlling one's hand temperature often requires long practice and repeated visits to a treatment center. Even then, many migraine sufferers would get little initial improvement. Most would get even less sustained benefit. For all but the most severely afflicted Group One sufferers, the time, inconvenience, and cost might seem to outweigh the highly uncertain outcome.

Other headache therapies, while perhaps more practical, fail to meet the test of safety. We have already had an unenthusiastic look at over-the-counter remedies, which cost Americans something like half a billion dollars a year and which have many unwanted and often dangerous side effects. Most of the commonly used prescription drugs have dangerous effects of their own.

Sansert (methysergide maleate tablets), for example, a relative of LSD, is often prescribed as a migraine preventative. Its action in the body is not fully understood, but it has the effect of reducing migraine cycles—making headaches come less often and last a shorter time. That is the good part. The bad part is that Sansert can inflict many kinds of damage. Either on initial exposure or after taking it for a period of time, some people experience drastic psychic effects. There may be hallucinations, bizarre physical sensations, inexplicable terrors. The drug can also cause fibrous thickening of tissues around the kidneys, in the lungs, and in the cardiac valves. Such thickening, when it happens, is extremely dangerous.

When migraine prevention fails, it is common to use an ergotamine preparation. (Cafergot is a commonly used combination of caffeine and ergotamine.) These drugs are vasoconstrictors. Their effect is to shrink the arteries whose dilation causes the pain of migraine. For best results, the patient must take them in what is called the "prodromal" phase of each migraine attack; that is, just before the headache sets in.

In the prodromal phase, the arteries constrict before starting to dilate, and it is this preliminary shrinking that causes the premigraine aura that many people experience—spots in front of the eyes, odd feelings around the head, sometimes numbness or tingling in an arm or hand, occasionally hallucinations. People who do not experience a well-defined prodromal aura, of course, never quite know when to take their medicine and may often take it when it is not necessary.

Ergotamine drugs bring on nausea and vomiting in many patients. For those who can take the drug more comfortably over a long period of time, there is the danger of ergotism. This disease causes anoxia—lack of sufficient oxygen carried by the blood—in fingers, toes, leg and heart muscles. In the extreme situation, one result can be gangrene, and another can be heart muscle damage (myocardial infarction).

Steroids (such as cortisone), another group of drugs used in migraine treatment, are anti-inflammatory agents. They help reduce congestion of blood vessels in the head. Among their unwanted side effects are weight gain and edema (swelling of tissues), which can lead to a moon-faced appearance or a "buffalo hump" in the back of the neck. They can also lead to a condition in which the bones become brittle, and they can produce body striae—lines of dark pigment in the skin.

These and other medicines are designed to attack the causes of headaches. In addition to them, of course, physicians prescribe drugs whose sole purpose is to relieve pain. Many such drugs are narcotics or narcotic-derivatives (such as Darvon), and they bring dangers of their own.

Often, such pain-relieving drugs will prevent normal functioning at home or at work. The patient is in a daze. His headache pain is dulled, but that is all he has gained. Instead of being incapacitated by pain, he is just as fully incapacitated by a narcotic.

The worst danger is addiction. The patient may become dependent on the drug, afraid to do without it. As tolerance develops, he must take it in ever larger quantities to produce the pain-deadening effect he wants. When he stops taking it, he may experience withdrawal symptoms—among which may be another headache. Fearing those withdrawal symptoms, fearing a return of his old pain, trying to cope with life stresses at the same time, he reaches a state in which he no longer feels he can live without the drug. He is hooked.

There is only one headache treatment I know of that fulfills the four criteria of effectiveness, safety, practicality, and low cost. *That treatment is auto-acupressure.*

CHAPTER

6

WHAT TO ASK—
AND TELL—
YOUR DOCTOR

THE HEADACHES of Group Three, the ones that are symptoms of serious disease or damage in the body, are not nearly as common as the vascular, tension, and sinus headaches of the other two groups. But it would be a mistake to assume offhand that your headaches do not fall into the danger-signal group. Even if your headaches are relatively mild and cause you only minor inconvenience, do not be fooled. The severity of a headache is no clue to its seriousness. Before attempting any self-treatment, including auto-acupressure, consult a physician and have him give you a thorough examination.

A medical doctor's examination is important even if you feel sure you have diagnosed your own head pain correctly. All the clues might point to common migraine, for example: the prodromal aura, the pain that begins behind one eye, the apparent connection with emotional upset, the family history of migraine, and so on. But self-diagnosis can be hazardous. It may or may not be true that you are suffering from migraine. Even if it is true, there is still the possibility that you have more than one kind of headache. I have seen double and even multiple types of headaches many times in my practice. One headache might partially mask the other, and the one that is masked might be a symptom of something dangerously wrong.

Because of this possible masking effect and because self-diagnosis is always unreliable, it is important that your doctor know everything about the state of your health. Tell him *all* the symptoms you have noticed, not just those you think are important. To emphasize this point, I would like to tell you the story of a woman who had four different types of headaches. One of them, a symptom of potentially serious trouble, might never have come to light if she had not described a dream.

Linda W. first consulted me because of tension and anxiety symptoms brought on by a difficult marriage that was heading for divorce. She was an attractive woman in her early forties. She had been a full-time wife and mother through most of her adult life, and, now that a divorce seemed imminent, she was trying to make plans for a new life of independence. She wanted to go back to secretarial school to relearn skills she had not used for about twenty years. But the tensions of her marriage got in her way.

She found herself unable to make even simple decisions, unable to work, easily upset, tired all the time for no apparent reason. Another symptom of this emotional turmoil was an almost constant tension headache, at the back of the neck and top of the head.

I helped her relieve these headaches partly through psychotherapy, which helped her control her constant state of anxiety, and partly with auto-acupressure. But then, a few months later, the divorce became final and a new set of symptoms appeared. She developed a cyclic pattern of depression. At the onset of menstruation each month she became irritable and unhappy, full of dark forebodings and thoughts about suicide. The depression was accompanied by a penetrating, throbbing pain in one side of her head—a classic migraine, apparently brought on by a combination of hormonal and emotional factors. When I prescribed antidepressant medication to be taken during these dark periods, the depression cycles were ameliorated and so were the headaches.

Not long after that, she began to experience another kind of headache. It seemed to be of migraine type. The pain was accompanied by sweating, weakness, and dizziness. But these headaches appeared to have no connection with her menstrual cycle. They occurred in a seemingly random pattern. "They're as likely to come at one time of month as another," she told me. "And they don't seem to have much connection with my emotional state. The only thing I've noticed is that they sometimes come on before lunch, or around ten or eleven at night when I'm getting ready for bed."

I asked, "Do you ever get one of these headaches

in the middle of the afternoon? Say around four o'clock?"

She nodded. "Yes, once or twice."

"If you have a headache and then eat a meal, does the headache get better?"

She thought for a while. "Yes," she said finally. "Come to think of it, eating does seem to make the headache go away."

It was a recognizable pattern: headaches three or four hours after meals, alleviated by the next meal. I ordered a five-hour glucose tolerance test that confirmed my suspicion. Her problem was functional hypoglycemia, a condition in which the blood sugar drops to abnormally low levels. Through complex bodily processes, this condition often brings on headaches. Even if your blood chemistry is normal, you may experience hypoglycemic or "hunger" headaches on days when you skip meals or try to get by on snacks. On such days, your blood sugar drops to levels that are not usual for you, and you end the day with an aching head. In Linda's case, the headaches were alleviated by a high-protein, low-carbohydrate diet that controlled her hypoglycemic condition.

Linda continued to consult me for psychotherapy after that. About a year later, during a therapy session, she told me about a dream. It was a Christmas scene. She was looking at a Christmas tree, and its lights were flashing on and off.

"By the way," she said casually, "that dream reminds me: I've been getting some headaches again. They often start when I see flashing lights."

This worried me. "Flashing lights?"

"Yes. At work, I have a fluorescent desk lamp that flickers, and it often seems to cause a headache. And when I'm driving home into the setting sun, I sometimes get a headache from seeing it dodge between buildings."

To a neurologist, those are symptoms to be taken seriously. I immediately ordered an electroencephalogram (EEG). The results were as I had feared. Linda was afflicted with a type of epilepsy.

Epilepsy can take many forms. It can remain hidden or can develop in middle or late adulthood, as in Linda's case. Sometimes, the first manifestation is an occasional headache—the equivalent of a seizure. If the illness is not treated, it may grow progressively more severe and may lead to grand mal seizures. Seizures are often brought on by flashing lights: a low sun seen through trees while driving along a road, or headlights of oncoming cars seen through a highway divider fence. Aircraft pilots sometimes develop seizures when they look at the sun shining through or reflecting off propeller blades, a problem that particularly troubles helicopter pilots.

I put Linda on antiepileptic medication. The flashing-light headaches ceased.

She had been through a harrowing few years. I am pleased to report that her story had a happy ending. While she was still in therapy, she and her divorced husband began seeing each other again. Today they are happily remarried.

Linda still has occasional migraine and tension headaches, which she controls perfectly with auto-acupressure, now that her hypoglycemia and epilepsy are fully under control. She has progressed from being a patient to being a disciple. She likes to demonstrate auto-acupressure to friends, and she preaches the advantage of the technique over drugs. But she always ends her informal lessons with an earnest injunction—one that she has learned from personal experience: *Never treat a headache until you know its cause.*

It is not my intention in this chapter to write a complete medical text on headaches and their causes. But I do want to make you fully aware of the potential danger of treating any headache too casually. Whether you treat it with pain-relieving drugs (from which I hope to wean you) or with auto-acupressure, it is never wise to do so without first getting a medical doctor's approval.

When you see your physician, he will want to know everything there is to know about your headaches —how and when they started, what they feel like, what other symptoms accompany them, and so on. The more information you can give him, and the more precise that information is, the better he can serve you. Thus, you will find it useful to review your own case before talking to him. Pay particular attention to the following factors.

ONSET: WHEN HEADACHES BEGAN

At what age did headaches first become a problem to you?

Did they begin so gradually that you cannot really pinpoint the onset, or was it more sudden? Headaches that begin suddenly after a lifetime of being relatively headache-free, or that abruptly grow more severe or more frequent, might indicate a tumor. On the other hand, if this is your history, do not alarm yourself by making a spot diagnosis. Common migraine headaches have been known to begin suddenly too, as in the case of George, the hard-driving executive with letdown migraine.

Was there a fever when your headaches began? Headaches that continue after a fever dies down may indicate various diseases such as meningitis or meningo-encephalitis.

At what time of year did the headaches start? If you can pinpoint the season, this may be a useful clue. For example, headaches that start in the fall may indicate that your body has developed an allergy to certain fall pollens. The body's chemistry is always changing, and a pollen that did not affect you last year might do so this year.

Has the pain been continuous or intermittently recurrent? Tension headaches are likely to be more constant than most other kinds, or else tend to recur at the same time of day.

((113))

PROGRESSION

Has the pain grown more severe over a period of time, or less severe? Or has there been no notable change? And how about the frequency? Do the headaches come more often than when they first began, or less often, or at about the same rate?

Many useful clues could be hidden in your answers to these questions. For instance, headache symptoms that rapidly grow more severe may indicate brain tumor, encephalitis, or malignant hypertension.

LOCATION

Where do you feel the pain? Is it generalized—seemingly all through your head? Or can you locate it more precisely? On one side, for instance, or in the temples?

We have already noted that tension headaches are usually felt around the top of the head and in the back of the neck, while migraines are often confined to one side or at least start on one side. Other kinds of headaches may be felt in other areas of the head. For instance, pain that seems confined to the temples may indicate temporal arteritis, a condition in which the internal artery walls thicken and interfere with blood supply. If the disease is not treated, it may progress to arteries within the brain.

NATURE OF PAIN

Does the pain seem to be on the surface or deep within your head? Is it sharp or dull? Does it have a "drilling" or knifelike quality, or does it feel more like pressure? Is there a definite throbbing, or is it constant?

These questions, too, can turn up important clues. Histamine cephalgia usually produces a penetrating, throbbing pain. The throbbing is caused by the regular expansion and contraction of dilated arteries as blood is pumped through them. Tension headaches, as well as some more serious ones, such as those caused by epilepsy or tumor, usually lack that pronounced throbbing quality and tend to be duller and more muted.

TIME PATTERNS

Tell your doctor anything you have noticed about the timing of your headaches. Is the pain with you constantly, or does it come and go? If it comes and goes, about how often does it return? Can you discern any pattern to the timing? We have already seen that seasonal patterns might be important, but how about daily patterns? When your headache returns, is it more likely to come at night, in the morning, before meals, after drinking alcoholic beverages?

Headaches that occur a few hours after meals may

indicate a hypoglycemic condition, as in Linda's case. If you often get a headache after a five-o'clock cocktail hour, this may mean you have a low tolerance for alcohol. Frequent end-of-day headaches may result from tension. Weekend headaches, as we saw in the last chapter, might be letdown migraine or might be caused by weekend social pressures.

PRECIPITATING FACTORS

The story of Annette J., the woman whose headaches came from eating Chinese food, illustrates that it can be useful to ask yourself what recurrent events in your life, if any, seem to be associated with the pain in your head. Think back to the last few times you had a headache and see if you can find a connection with something else, no matter how farfetched the connection might seem. Are your headaches often preceded or accompanied or followed by any particular event, any activity, any state of mind or body?

For instance, do you get headaches before, during, or after a menstrual period? Do you get them when you are tired? When you are hungry? After drinking? While driving? While playing golf or gardening? When you see flashing lights? When you smoke more than usual? When you take certain medicines? If you can think of any such connection, *however remote*, it may provide your doctor with a key to the puzzle.

ASSOCIATED SYMPTOMS

When your head hurts, what else happens? The associated symptoms that appear before, during, and after a headache often signal the kind of headache it is.

Watery eyes, runny nose, and a red, blotchy face often indicate histamine cephalgia. Pain in the face may point to neuralgia, while pain in the abdomen accompanying a headache can be a symptom of epilepsy. Abdominal pain also occurs sometimes with severe migraine. Other associated symptoms are nausea, vomiting, and profuse sweating. Pain, weakness, or tingling in the limbs or face may indicate migraine, or may be symptoms of a more serious vascular disorder in the brain.

Many visual changes can be associated with migraine: blurring, inability to focus on close work, blind spots, bright spots or "stars," sometimes even hallucinations. Olfactory hallucinations—smelling strange odors that are not really there—sometimes go along with migraine, or may be a symptom of epilepsy. Auditory hallucinations—hearing nonexistent sounds, voices, music—can point to temporal lobe epilepsy. Dizziness and vertigo might be symptoms of high blood pressure. Periods of confusion and speech problems—difficulty with pronunciation or with finding words—can accompany head pain in many conditions, among them migraine, epilepsy, and brain tumor.

QUICK HEADACHE RELIEF
WITHOUT DRUGS

WHAT MAKES HEADACHES WORSE?

If you find that certain conditions or bodily positions usually make your pain more severe, this information may help your doctor in his diagnosis.

For instance, does the pain seem to increase when you cough, sneeze, or wear a tight collar? That symptom might point to brain tumor. A tumor causes pain mainly by increasing intracranial pressure (pressure within the head), and anything such as a sneeze, which momentarily increases the pressure still more, tends to make the pain more severe.

Or does your head hurt more when you lie down? That is often a symptom of common migraine.

WHAT RELIEVES THE PAIN?

Similarly, useful clues might lie in the facts about what alleviates the pain.

If the pain seems to diminish quickly when you lie down, then it is probable that your headaches are not caused by any malfunction inside your head. They may be tension headaches, for instance, or the result of a mild, transitory fever.

If you seem able to cure your headaches simply by eating food, the problem may be hypoglycemia.

Your doctor will also want to know what drugs, if any, you have been taking to relieve the pain. He will want to know, too, how much of the drug or drugs you take to control the pain on a typical headache day, and whether the amount you seem to need has increased over the years.

FAMILY HISTORY

I have already mentioned that a tendency toward migraine headaches seems to be inheritable, at least to some extent. Certain other headache-associated diseases and tendencies may also be handed down genetically from one generation to another. If you know of such a problem in your family tree, it is important that you let your doctor know about it.

Tell him if your family has a history of mental illness, or of neurological diseases, such as epilepsy, or of hypertension, brain tumor, or congenital aneurysm (a tendency for blood-vessel walls to have weak places and to develop balloonlike swellings at those spots). Also tell him if your family has an unusually high incidence of *any* disease, whether or not that disease *seems* to have anything to do with headaches.

PERSONALITY FACTORS

We have seen that emotional stresses can often trigger headaches or can become tangled up with various bodily mechanisms that lead to them, or, in the case of tension headaches, can be the prime cause. Before talking to your physician, try to make a calm and realistic appraisal of your life, its stresses, and your personal reaction to them.

Did your headaches begin in a period when you were particularly upset about something? Do they now seem to come on when you are feeling depressed, angry, overworked? Your doctor may find it helpful to know if there are serious emotional problems of any kind in your life, for example, problems involving your job or lack of one, your marriage or other man-woman relationships, your social life, your relationship with your own or your spouse's parents, your relationship with your children.

It will also be important to tell him what drugs you are taking, if any—in addition to those you may have been taking to relieve headache pain. For example, do you regularly use sleeping pills or tranquilizers? Are you a regular user of any kind of mood-changing drug, including alcohol?

If you do take such a drug, even a seemingly mild one and even in what you feel are moderate amounts, try to assess its importance in your life. Ask yourself whether you *depend* on it to any degree in helping you cope with life and its stresses. And think back to the last few times you had a headache. Did the pain develop at a time when you neglected to take the drug, or were you trying to do without it, or for some reason were you unable to get your usual intake?

It is important to be honest with yourself and your

physician in answering these questions. Even some supposedly nonaddictive, nonprescription drugs can weave themselves so tightly into men's and women's lives that it is hard to banish them. If you have been taking a sleeping pill or tranquilizer or "nervous-tension reliever" for a span of time, with or without a doctor's prescription, you may have developed a state of dependency. On any day when you take less than your usual amount, you may experience withdrawal symptoms—among which may be a headache.

OTHER ESSENTIAL DATA

Finally, tell your doctor about any of these significant health factors that might apply in your case:

• Serious bodily injury, especially head injuries that may have happened within the last five years. It is perfectly possible to injure your head, even to the extent of fracturing your skull, and not realize for months or even years that any serious damage was done. Headache and other symptoms may turn up a long time later.

One possible result of a blow on the head is a hematoma, a swelling filled with clotted blood. A hematoma can form under the outer covering of the brain (subdural) or outside it (extradural). If it is not treated, it can lead to headache and other, more serious problems.

• Surgery you have undergone, especially recent surgery. This includes minor surgery such as tooth extraction. Any surgery around the head—surgery of the eyes, nose, ears, teeth—can trigger headaches in some people, and the headaches will sometimes continue long after the surgical wound seems completely healed. Also, anesthetics and anti-infection drugs such as penicillin can trigger headaches by causing allergic reactions.

• Recent changes in diet, or any unusual new element of your diet. For instance, some high carbohydrate diets can cause the blood sugar to fall to relatively low levels, and the result can be hypoglycemic "hunger" headaches. Even if that does not happen, weight-loss diets can cause fatigue because the body is not getting all the food energy it is accustomed to. Fatigue can lead to irritability, which in turn can lead to tension headaches.

Your doctor may want details of your diet even if you eat normal amounts of common foods. He might suspect that you have some kind of food allergy, for instance, as did Annette, the temporary victim of CRS. Prepare for his questions now by asking yourself whether headaches seem to come on after eating certain foods.

• History of any fainting spell, blackout (a period "lost" from your memory), or convulsion. Even if such an event happened far back in your past and has never been repeated, it might indicate some neurological problem that still exists and that may now be contributing to your headaches.

• Use of tobacco. Smoking can cause headaches in

some people, for nicotine and other elements in tobacco smoke can be toxic. In other people, smoking can exacerbate vascular or other problems that might not otherwise cause much difficulty.

• Drugs and medicines you are taking or have recently taken for any reason. I have already mentioned pain-killing and mood-changing drugs, but it is possible that others will turn out to have a bearing on your case. Almost any drug can produce an allergic reaction or can upset your body chemistry in some other way. Tell your doctor about anything you have been taking, including nonprescription drugs, such as cold remedies, cough medicines, laxatives.

• Unusual sun sensitivity. This might indicate a metabolic disease called porphyria. Among its common symptoms are headaches.

• General-system diseases that you may have had. Many such diseases—rheumatic fever, for example, or measles—can leave various kinds of long-term or permanent damage behind.

When you have given your doctor all the information you can, he will undoubtedly give you a physical examination, and it is possible he will order some special tests to help his diagnosis. He may want you to have certain blood tests, for example, and he may order skull X rays, an EEG, or a brain scan if some of the clues he has picked up lead him to think these are necessary.

Statistically, the odds are high that you will walk

out of his office with the knowledge that no serious illness or damage lies behind your headaches. Even if there is an underlying cause that he feels should be and can be treated, he may still recommend that you use a nonprescription analgesic or auto-acupressure to control the pain.

One way or the other, you are about to discover the benefits of drug-free pain relief. It is time to get you started.

CHAPTER

7

**THE ANATOMY
OF HEADACHE
RELIEF:
PRESSURE
POINTS**

WE NOW COME to the heart of the matter. I am going to teach you how to banish the pain of headache simply by using your thumbs. If you feel it took us a while to get to this point, I am sorry; but I must emphasize again that I am a conscientious physician and I could not, in fairness to *your* health, give you these instructions without the necessary background and cautionary counsel that precede them.

Now, since I have promised to get right down to cases, I will begin by saying quite simply that there are eight pressure points on the body for relieving the vascular and muscle-contraction headaches of the most common type (Group One). They are arranged in *four pairs:* near the eyes, on the neck, near the thumbs, and at the wrists.

In this chapter, I will explain where the points are, with words and illustrations. In the next chapter, I will tell you how to apply pressure to these points. It is important that you locate the four pairs on your body with precision and press them in exactly the right way. If you do not, nothing much will happen, although you certainly will not be any worse off than before. I am emphasizing the need for precision on your part because even a seemingly slight deviation from the right spot, or a seemingly trivial mistake in the way you press, could mean that your headache stays with you.

All eight of the points are located at places where headache-related nerves come within reach of manipulation from the outside. At other places in your body, these same nerves are hidden behind bone or buried in masses of muscle or other tissue. At the eight pressure points, the nerves emerge and are accessible to pressure on the skin surface.

The nerve areas are not large. It is quite easy to miss them. Each pressure point (except for one newly discovered pair) has been defined after hundreds or thousands of years of empirical observation and confirmed by my own neurophysiological studies. Each is the point where the given nerve or nerves are most readily available for pressure. When you press correctly, you press directly on the nerve. If you are even a quarter-inch off the center of the target, there may not be enough pressure on the nerve and you will get disappointing results.

I have said before that there is no agreement on

((128))

how acupressure (or acupuncture, for that matter) works. But some oversimplify the process by thinking that when you press on a nerve, you temporarily "overload" the pain interpretation centers with impulses. When you stop pressing, the pain circuit is, in effect, inoperative or "jammed" for a while. It can no longer interpret or reinforce headache pain signals clearly. The result is that your sensation of head pain diminishes or simply stops.

Do not be confused by the fact that, although the pain is in your head, I am asking you to press your hand or neck. The pain message travels through your complex nervous system. Pain messages can be "intercepted" at specific points where the nerves that come close to the surface of your body interconnect with specific pain-perception pathways in the autonomic and central nervous systems.

Here's another way of trying to understand how acupressure relieves pain. Think of it in terms of a feedback system, like the thermostat that regulates the temperature of your home. When everything is working properly, the thermostat turns on your furnace or electric heating elements whenever it senses that the air temperature has fallen below the setting, and then it turns the heat back off when the temperature has risen slightly above that mark.

But suppose something goes wrong with the sys-

---

tem. The temperature rises above the setting, the thermostat fails to sense the increase and the furnace keeps running. An imbalance exists that is roughly analogous to the nervous-system imbalance that can bring on a headache.

Perhaps a part of the thermostat mechanism is blocked or stuck. One way to make it come unstuck might be to overload it temporarily. Hold a lighted table lamp under it for a few seconds. The thermostat *at last* senses that the temperature has gone far above the setting. The overload makes the stuck mechanism spring loose, and the furnace receives the signal to turn itself off.

The thermostat-furnace analogy is very inexact, of course. I do not present it as a medical explanation of the remarkable effects of acupressure, but simply as one way to visualize what happens. My main point is that, no matter how you choose to visualize the process or what analogy you use, acupressure works by feeding impulses into nerves that are involved in the bodily imbalance whose symptom is headache. You must work directly on those nerves, by locating the four pairs of pressure points carefully and exactly.

One way to tell when you are on the right spot is that it will feel extremely sensitive when you press it. Even when you do not have a headache, the pressure points feel more tender than other points nearby. When you do have a headache, the points are decidedly more tender—so much so, sometimes, that merely touching them causes an odd sensation. Not everyone feels this as a sensation of pain—although almost all of my patients are startled by the sensation when I first employ acupressure on them—it is always, at least, a somewhat unpleasant, uncomfortable feeling. This also applies to *auto*-acupressure, the use of the technique on oneself. Not everyone has the courage to inflict real pain on himself, even if only for a few seconds. However, all except the most timid soon enough come to realize that seconds of pain are preferable to hours of headaches.

The "unpleasant feeling" is something like the sensation you get when you hit the funny bone at the back of your elbow. That peculiar sensation does not come from hitting a bone but from hitting an exposed nerve in that area of the elbow joint. The unpleasant feeling —partly pain, partly numbness, partly a sense of tingling—can travel all the way down your arm and into your hand.

Thus it is with the headache pressure points. When you have located a point correctly and are pressing on it in the right way, the sensation will seem to travel beyond that one point.

As I describe the points to you, try to locate them with your thumbnails. Dig your nails *hard* into the indicated loci, exploring until you find the sensitive spot in each case. In the rare case of unusually sharp or rigid thumbnails, the nails should be rounded to prevent penetration of the skin.

If you have trouble finding the points in a period when you do not have a headache, wait until the next headache strikes and then try again. In all likelihood, you will find the points easily at that time. They will definitely be tender, if not painful. If the headache seems confined to one side of your head, you will often, but not always find the four points on that side of your body more tender than those on the other side.

The Group One headaches, meaning the common type as described earlier, respond to pressure on two pairs of *main* points (on the head) and two pairs of *accessory* points (on the hands). Do not worry about this distinction just yet. I will explain the reasons for it in the next chapter. For now, I just want you to locate the four pairs of points on your own body.

In each case, I will give the Chinese name of the point, as set down in traditional Chinese practice, and the English translation of that name. I will do this more for fun than for any other reason. There is no need for you to remember the Chinese names unless you find them appealing. These Chinese names are more like poetry than medical science. Poetry will not help you relieve your headache, but you may find that it relieves the somewhat grim, humorless quality of headache treatment. (There is nothing funny about headaches, of course, except to people who do not get them.) So if the Chinese names help lighten your mood and restore your optimism, by all means use them. For the sake of clarity, I will use my own English-language designations for the remainder of the book.

In case you do want to use the Chinese words, I will give you some guidance in pronouncing them. These pronunciation guides are by no means exact, for many sounds in the Chinese language are hard to render in English. To complicate the problem further, there are many Chinese dialects. A given word may be pronounced in many different ways. Thus, the best I can do is give you suggestions about pronunciation.

Here are the four pairs of Group One pressure points. Learn them well. They could change your life.

HEAD 1: THE FIRST MAIN POINT

Chinese name: *Tai Yang*
Suggested pronunciation: *tie yang*
Translation: Great Solar
Affected nerves: Divisions of the trigeminal nerve associated with the areas above eyes (ophthalmic division) and upper jaw (maxillary division). Also, temporal branches of the facial nerve associated with muscles in the head and face.

((**133**))

QUICK HEADACHE RELIEF
WITHOUT DRUGS

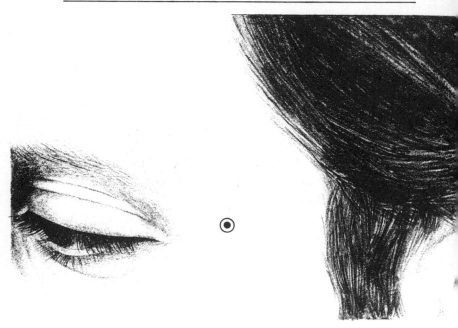

HOW TO FIND HEAD 1—LEFT SIDE. *Note that the point is not as far back as the large hollow of the temple. It is one finger's breadth from the bony ridge at the outer corner of your eye. When you find and press it correctly, you will stimulate an exposed nerve.*

How to find it: First find a point halfway between the outer corner of your eye and the outer end of your eyebrow. Your finger should be on a ridge of bone, the outer edge of the eye socket in your skull. (The use of a mirror is helpful the first time you locate this point. After that, you will be able to put your finger, or rather your thumb, right on it.) Now move one finger's breadth

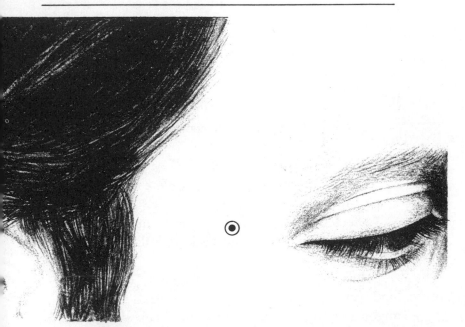

HOW TO FIND HEAD 1—RIGHT SIDE. *It is important to press both Head 1 points simultaneously, as will be explained later. Before pressing with full force, probe around until you hit a point that gives you a "funny bone" feeling.*

back toward your ear, and you will find a small depression. This is Head 1.

One mistake many people make when hunting for this point is to move too far back from the eye-and-eyebrow starting place. Go *only* a finger's breadth, no more. If you are as far back as the large hollow of the temple, you have gone too far.

Head 1 is a newly discovered point, apparently not known to traditional acupuncture, let alone auto-acupressure.

HEAD 2: THE SECOND MAIN POINT

Chinese name: *Feng Chih*
Suggested pronunciation: *feng chee*
Translation: Wind Pond
Affected nerves: Greater and minor occipital nerves, associated with the neck and the back at the base of the head.

How to find it: First find the bony ridge just behind your ear—the mastoid bone. Next find the big muscular groove at midpoint in the back of your neck. Halfway between these two places, on each side of your neck, you will find another, smaller groove between two large muscles. When you have located this smaller groove, run your thumbnail up it until you come to the base of your skull. Push inward and upward hard, into the groove and against the bone. This is Head 2.

If you have trouble finding that smaller muscle groove, it may help to tense your neck muscles. Do this by sitting on a hard chair, leaning forward and looking at your toes. This makes your posterior neck muscles hold up the weight of your head, tenses them, and makes the groove more pronounced.

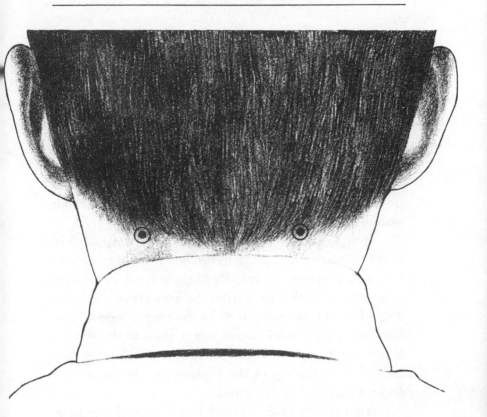

HOW TO FIND HEAD 2. *As is true of Head 1, this is a pair of points that must be pressed simultaneously for the best results. The two points are right under and against the base of the skull, in the two small muscular grooves at the back of your neck.*

QUICK HEADACHE RELIEF
WITHOUT DRUGS

Chinese name: *Ho Ku*
Suggested pronunciation: *ho koo*
Translation: Connecting the Valleys
Affected nerves: Superficial branches of the radial nerve and deep palmar muscle branches of the ulnar nerve. These are complexes of cervico-spinal nerves that travel up the arm to link with the autonomic nervous system and spinal cord in the neck.

How to find it: The point is in the triangle of flesh between your thumb and index finger on the back of the hand. It is near the middle of the second metacarpal bone—the bone that runs from the knuckle of the index finger back to the wrist. It is on the thumb side of that bone and closer to the index finger than to the thumb. When the thumb and index finger are held together, Hand 1 is on the top of the highest spot in the web of flesh on the back of the hand.

A good way to find Hand 1 is to spread one hand out so that the web of the thumb is stretched. Straighten the other thumb and bring it pointing upward to the middle of the stretched web. The web should run across the first joint of the straightened thumb. In other words, the web runs along the fold of skin just below the ball of the thumb where the tip of the thumb bends. Now bend the thumb over toward the web on the back of the opposite hand until the tip of the thumb touches the fleshy web.

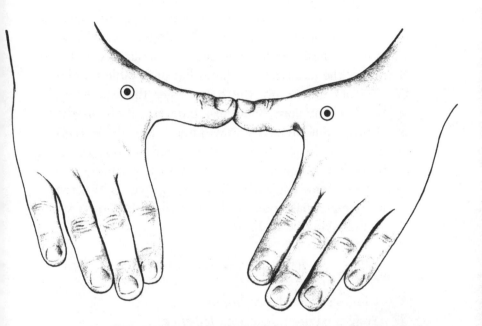

HOW TO FIND HAND 1. *Again, this is a pair of points—one on each hand. Note that the point is against the second metacarpal (index finger) bone. When you probe for it, probe inward toward the main body of the hand, not outward against the thumb bone.*

Push downward and inward with your thumbnail, as though trying to push beneath the muscle. Move the thumbnail back and forth along the web, a fraction of an inch at a time. You will finally get to a tender spot. You are pressing on nerves. You have found Hand 1.

A mistake some people make in trying to locate Hand 1 is to probe along the index finger's tendon instead of the flesh next to the second metacarpal bone. If you lay the palm of your hand flat on a tabletop and lift the four fingers up, the four ridges that stand out on the back of your hand are tendons. Push on the index-finger tendon, and you will find it flexible. It gives when you push. If you now slide your pushing finger off that tendon, toward the thumb, you will hit something solid—something with little or no give. That is the second metacarpal bone, and you will find Hand 1 on the thumb side of that bone.

HAND 2: THE SECOND ACCESSORY POINT

Chinese name: *Lieh Chueh*
Suggested pronunciation: *lee chee*
Translation: Extreme Shortcoming
Affected nerves: Lateral antibrachial cutaneous nerve and branches of the radial nerve. These nerves also travel up the arm to join the cervical plexus of nerves and the autonomic nervous system in the neck.

How to find it: Spread both hands and put the two thumb webs together crosswise, so that the fingers of one hand are over the back of the other. Move the upper index finger down so that it rests on the radial side (thumb side) of your wrist. Where the fingertip or the ball of the finger comes to rest, you will find a protuberance of bone. This is the styloid process at the

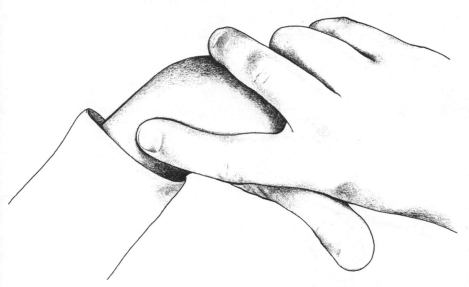

HOW TO FIND HAND 2—LEFT WRIST. *With the two thumbs web-to-web as shown, the index finger rests on a bony protuberance in the left wrist. Slightly above the protuberance is the sensitive Hand 2 point, where a nerve comes close to the surface.*

end of the radius, the bone at the thumb side of your forearm. Two fingers' width above the styloid process you will find a small depression, and in that depression is Hand 2.

People's hands and fingers differ in relative length, so you may not find Hand 2 immediately with the finger-pointing approach. Another way to find it is to spread your thumb out and back as far as it will go. Two long tendons will stand out, and in between these tendons,

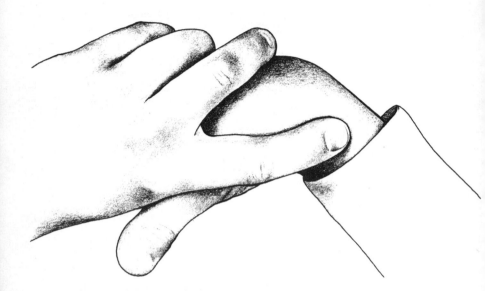

HOW TO FIND HAND 2—RIGHT WRIST. *For many, this is a hard point to find. Probe for it carefully on both wrists. Then test your accuracy with a preliminary dig of your thumbnail to see if you produce a tingling sensation.*

where they vanish into the wrist, will be a hollow space. This space is sometimes called the "anatomical snuff-box" because, in centuries past, people put pinches of snuff into it and sniffed from it. Immediately above the anatomical snuffbox is the styloid process, and two fingers' width above that is the small depression you are hunting for.

To test the point, push downward on it with your thumbnail. There should be a tender feeling, with a sensation of pain or pressure spreading up your arm or into your hand.

I would suggest that you review the information conveyed in this chapter and, in fact, study it and experiment with it until you have a good "fix" on the location of these four pressure points. Once you have done this, you are ready for the next lesson on how to use the pressure points.

CHAPTER
8

HOW TO USE THE PRESSURE POINTS

THERE ARE EFFECTIVE ways to apply auto-acupressure, and there are ineffective ways. This chapter is, in essence, a manual of effective techniques: how and when to press the Group One points to obtain the most effective relief from headache pain. The efficacy of these techniques has been demonstrated not only with patients of varied backgrounds, but also with physician volunteers at national medical meetings.

I will begin with some general instructions that apply to all the Group One points. (Most of these instructions will also apply to the Sinus points we will consider in Chapter Nine). Then I'll give you directions that apply specifically to each of the Group One points.

GENERAL DIRECTIONS

Always press with your thumbnail, not the ball of your thumb or the fleshy tip. The object is to apply *hard*, even painful, pressure on a small area. Here are my specific instructions:

• The thumb should be bent so that the two joints form a right angle. In this position, your thumb can exert a surprisingly powerful force.

• Press hard enough to make the point hurt. Do not worry: The pain will not last long. Compared with the length of time your headache might last, the duration of acupressure pain is trivial. Remember what I said in a previous chapter: that you can think of acupressure as a process in which you temporarily overload a nerve pathway with impulses. Unavoidably, this overloading hurts. If you do not make it hurt, you will get unsatisfactory results or none at all.

One way to look at it is that you are striking an excellent bargain. By enduring a short period of sharp pain at the pressure points, you are getting out of a long period—Who knows how long?—of misery from the pain in your head. As one of my patients remarked, "It's like spending a dollar and getting a thousand back."

• Press each point for fifteen to thirty seconds. (Does the bargain begin to sound better and better?)

• If you find that steady pressure gives you adequate relief, that is fine. However, some people find that an alternating technique works better for them—particularly when the headache is unusually severe or the pressure points are very tender. This alternating method is one of rhythmic off-and-on pressure.

In this technique, you increase and decrease the pressure once or twice a second throughout the fifteen-to-thirty-second period. *Push* hard, then ease off, then *push* again.

Not only does this help when your head hurts severely and you are reluctant to touch it, but also many people find that the off-and-on technique enables them to apply the necessary hard pressure more effectively. For some, pressing steadily on a point for a quarter or half minute is too much of a demand on the thumb and hand muscles. Anyway, the tendency for most people who apply steady pressure is to press forcefully in the beginning but then gradually slacken off without realizing it.

• Always press *both* points in any given pair. The points on your head and neck (Head 1 and Head 2) can be pressed as pairs, using your two hands simultaneously. Those on your hands and wrists (Hand 1 and Hand 2) must obviously be pressed one after the other, since you have only two hands to work with. But in all cases, be sure you never neglect one half of a pair.

This is important even if your headache is definitely one-sided, and even if the pressure points on that side are decidedly the more tender. If you press only one side, your headache may shift to the other side.

I have emphasized the need to push hard with the thumbnail, so as to put forceful pressure on a small, defined point. Now I want to make sure I have not overemphasized it. It is *not* necessary to press so hard that you injure the skin. And *do not* sharpen your thumbnails or reinforce them with plastic nail extenders. An ordinary blunt thumbnail, pushed hard enough to affect the underlying nerves but not hard enough to puncture the skin, will do the trick.

I was concerned about the possibility that patients might injure their skin when I first began teaching auto-acupressure. Many patients told me that they pushed harder as time went by. They grew more adept with the technique, more confident, more enthusiastic about its remarkable effects. Thus, after a few weeks or months, they found themselves pressing less timidly than when they had started. I was concerned that some of them would get too enthusiastic and apply so much pressure that they would do damage to their skin.

In practice, this has not happened. I have known only one patient who overdid the pressure to that extent. It seems that most people gradually increase pressure over a span of time until they reach the point of "enough," and there they instinctively stop.

Today, after years of working with the technique and observing how people use it, I am more concerned about your applying too *little* pressure than too *much*. What you must do is experiment with your own headaches, which, as I have said before, are never exactly like anybody else's headaches. It may turn out that relatively light pressure is enough for you, while someone else may need a good deal more force to make the technique effective. "Enough" pressure, of course, is the amount that relieves your headaches. When your headache is relieved, stop. Increase the pressure no more.

POINT-ORDER DIRECTIONS

Start by pressing the accessory points, Hand 1 (near the thumbs) and Hand 2 (on the wrists). This reduces the pain in your head and makes the main points near your temples and on your neck less tender. You will then find it easier to press them with the necessary force.

• Of the two accessory points, Hand 1 is generally the more effective, and it is also easier to find. So you will usually find it sufficient to use the first accessory point alone and ignore Hand 2. Use Hand 2 when you cannot use Hand 1 for some reason.

If you have by chance injured your hand, for instance, you may not be able to get at the first accessory point on that hand, or you may find it so tender that you cannot press it hard enough to affect your headache. In that case, use the wrist points. There is also the possibility, of course, of enlisting the services of a willing accomplice.

• There should be an appreciable lessening of head pain when you press the accessory points properly. In some people, the pain seems to vanish completely with pressure on the accessory points alone. But if it is merely reduced, you should go on to press the main points. If you do not, the headache may return to its original severity.

Late in 1975, I gave a lecture at the Cook County (Chicago) Graduate School of Medicine. My audience was composed of physicians. I convinced two skeptical psychiatrists that acupressure works. In both cases I banished their headaches with pressure on Hand 1 alone, using the rhythmic off-and-on technique.

That first accessory point, Hand 1, is indeed an effective one—so much so that it seems almost magical to many who try it for the first time. Still, do not stop there. For longer-lasting relief, ordinarily, you must press the main points too.

• Press both pairs of main points: first Head 1 (near the temple) and then Head 2 (at the back of the neck). Pressure on Head 1 alone may give you instant and apparently complete relief, but the headache may return if you neglect Head 2.

• *Do not* use the *Hand* points if you are pregnant. Even though the technique is safer and more natural than loading your body with pain-killing pills, there is a suspicion in some medical quarters that it might lead to miscarriage or other complications in pregnancy. The evidence to support this is very slight and not at all conclusive, but as long as even a hint of danger exists, I would rather have you avoid it.

As a matter of fact, there is much stronger evidence that aspirin causes some pregnancy complications. A research team in Australia recently reported finding a high incidence of problems in women who took significant amounts of aspirin while they were pregnant. As against light or moderate users of aspirin, heavy users are more likely to have problems such as anemia, hemorrhage, and urinary tract infection. Moreover, the gestation period for heavy users tends to be longer, and there are more likely to be complications in delivery. There is also evidence that heavy use of aspirin increases the chances of stillbirth.

Indeed, many physicians have long advocated that a pregnant woman should be cautious about taking *any* drug, for *any* reason. Not enough is known about the effects of drugs on the unborn baby. Nor is enough known about the mechanisms by which drugs do or do not pass from the mother's body to the baby's.

From this point of view, using the auto-acupressure main points would seem to be a safer way to attack headaches than aspirin or any other drug. But if you are pregnant, or suspect you might be, ask your medical doctor for his advice before attempting any self-treatment method, whether it is acupressure, aspirin, or anything else.

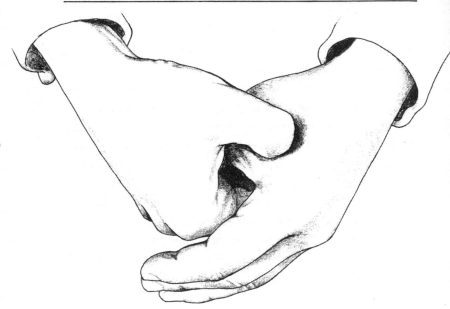

HOW TO PRESS HAND 1—LEFT HAND. *The secret is hard pressure with the thumbnail. Note that the thumb is bent into a right angle—a position in which it can exert the strongest force. Use the fingers for leverage and squeeze hard. Don't be timid.*

POINT-BY-POINT DIRECTIONS

HAND 1

This point, like all the others, must be pressed *firmly* with your thumbnail for good results. To make sure your thumb has the right leverage, put the fingers of that hand under the palm of the hand being pressed. Then squeeze with the fingers as you press your thumb-

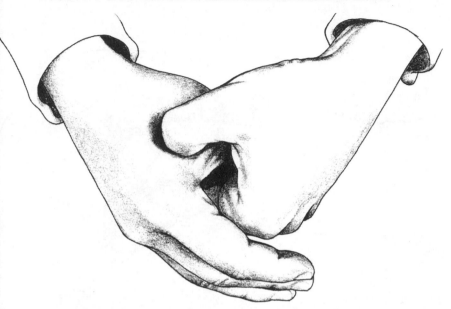

HOW TO PRESS HAND 1—RIGHT HAND. *When you do it correctly, the sensation "travels" beyond the pressure point itself. Obviously, you can't press both of your hands simultaneously, but if you're helping a friend, you'll get better results that way.*

nail into the point on the back of the hand.

The thumbnail should press near the middle of the second metacarpal bone on the back of the hand, in the web between the thumb and index finger. As I have said, the point will feel peculiarly tender when you are properly on target. If it does not feel tender, that means either that you are not pressing hard enough or that you have missed the target. Explore the center of the web between the thumb and index finger with your thumbnail until you hit the tender place, and then press *hard*.

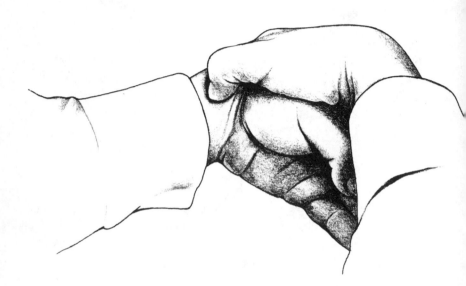

HOW TO PRESS HAND 2—LEFT HAND. *The thumb is bent to a right angle. Its strength is reinforced by answering pressure from the fingers on the other side of your hand or wrist. Press hard enough to make the point hurt—but no longer than thirty seconds.*

HAND 2

As with Hand 1, you can increase the leverage of your thumbnail on this point by putting your fingers

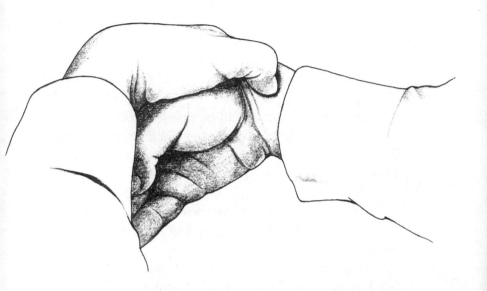

HOW TO PRESS HAND 2—RIGHT HAND. *Always press both points in each pair—even with a one-sided headache. If steady pressure seems too painful, use alternating pressure.*

under the heel of the hand being pressed. Your thumbnail should be pressing downward on the bony area, two fingers' breadth above the styloid process (which, you will recall, is the protuberance of bone at the top of the anatomical snuffbox). Dig the nail in firmly, as though trying to push it into your wrist, and squeeze hard with your fingers to oppose the pressure of your thumb.

QUICK HEADACHE RELIEF
WITHOUT DRUGS

HEAD 1

If you wear glasses, you must remove them to gain access to this point.

The Head 1 pair should be pressed simultaneously, with your two thumbs opposing each other. To gain the right leverage, start by clasping your fingers in front of your forehead, with your palms toward your face. Pull your two thumbs back into the bent position in which they can exert the most force. Now explore with your thumbnails until you find the tender Head 1 points.

Depending on the relation of the width of your head to the size of your hands, you may find it necessary to adjust the way in which your fingers are clasped as you put your thumbnails into the pressure points. The clasp should be comfortably firm—not so tight that you can't work your thumbs into position, but not loose either. One index finger should rest firmly against your forehead. You now have your head in a caliperlike grip, and it will be easy to exert all the pressure you need.

Push the two thumbnails hard into the pressure points, exerting a squeezing force with your hands and fingers. You may find the pain fairly sharp for the first second or two, but it will subside. Be sure you maintain steady or rhythmic off-and-on pressure for at least a full fifteen seconds.

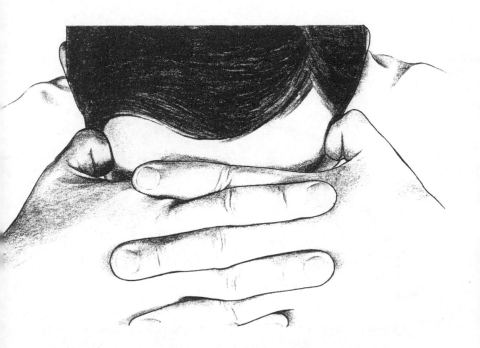

HOW TO PRESS HEAD 1. *The fingers are interlocked so that you can hold your head in a strong, caliper-like grip. Again, notice the bent thumbs. If you try acupressure with your thumbs straight, you simply will not be able to generate enough force.*

QUICK HEADACHE RELIEF
WITHOUT DRUGS

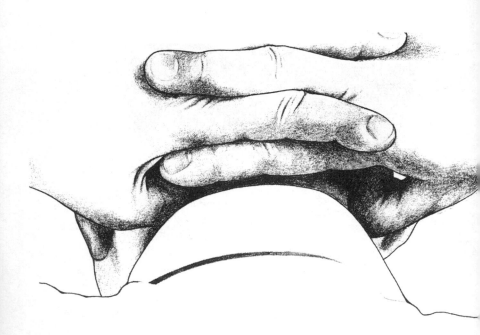

HOW TO PRESS HEAD 2. *The fingers are behind your head or on top, depending on how you feel most comfortable. Push your thumbnails inward against your neck and upward aaginst the base of your skull, hard enough to stretch the skin of the neck.*

HEAD 2

Put your two hands behind your ears, with the fingers clutching the top of your head. The thumbnail pressure in Head 2 should be inward against the neck and upward against the base of the skull. Push hard enough so that the skin at the back of the neck stretches.

As I said, people differ in the relative sizes of their fingers. When pressing Head 2, you may find that you are more comfortable and can exert pressure most easily when your fingertips do not quite touch on the top of your head. Or, if your fingers are longer, you may find it helps to interlace the fingertips. Do it either way—just as long as the pressure is forceful.

And now, in the next few chapters, we will learn how to relieve the pain of the more complicated and more damaging types of headaches, particularly the sinus headache. Fortunately, these are less common than those of the Group One type. If you get sinus headaches, you need to know the information presented in the next chapter.

CHAPTER
9

THE
SINUS
HEADACHES

I HAVE GIVEN sinus headaches this chapter and the next to themselves because I want you to take them very, very seriously. If a physician diagnoses your headaches as being caused wholly or partly by a problem in the sinuses, you should put yourself in his care and consult him regularly during all the time you are using auto-acupressure for the pain. Auto-acupressure can relieve the pain, but it will not combat sinus disease itself. The disease may or may not be dangerous, but it makes no sense to take chances.

I met an American woman living in Hong Kong who had been given acupuncture treatments for sinus headaches. The treatments almost completely alleviated the pain, and she was well satisfied with them—until an alert physician discovered that the disease, in this case bacterial sinusitis, had progressed to a very dangerous point. The sinusitis had eroded part of the sinus bone, and the infection was rapidly making its way to her brain. Her life was rescued by emergency neurosurgery and antibiotics.

Whether you use acupressure or aspirin or any other pain-relieving approach for your sinus headache, you are taking grave risks if you do so without also having a medical doctor treat the underlying disease.

The so-called sinus headaches spring from various kinds of allergies, infections, and other problems in a group of bony cavities called the paranasal sinuses.

These cavities make the skull lighter than it would otherwise be, and they also serve to give resonance to the voice.

In most people, there are four pairs of paranasal sinus cavities. They are connected with the nose and are lined with extensions of the same mucous membrane that lines the nasal passages.

The *frontal sinuses* are above the eyes and the root of the nose. They give rise to the ridge or prominence between your eyebrows. In some animals—elephants and owls, for instance—they are proportionately much bigger than in man, and they give those animals a bulging forehead and a reputation for braininess. In man, they vary widely in size and shape. They are usually very small or nonexistent in a newborn baby, and they develop gradually and irregularly as the individual grows. In about fifteen percent of men and women, only one frontal sinus develops, and about five percent have no frontal sinuses at all.

The *sphenoid sinuses* and *ethmoid sinuses* are lower in the skull, near the eyes and behind the cheekbones. They do not vary as much in size or shape as do the frontal sinuses. The sphenoid sinus begins to develop at about three years of age and does not reach adult size until adolescence.

The *maxillary sinuses* are farther back in the skull, above the back teeth. When they are diseased, they may cause pain that is mistakenly felt as a toothache.

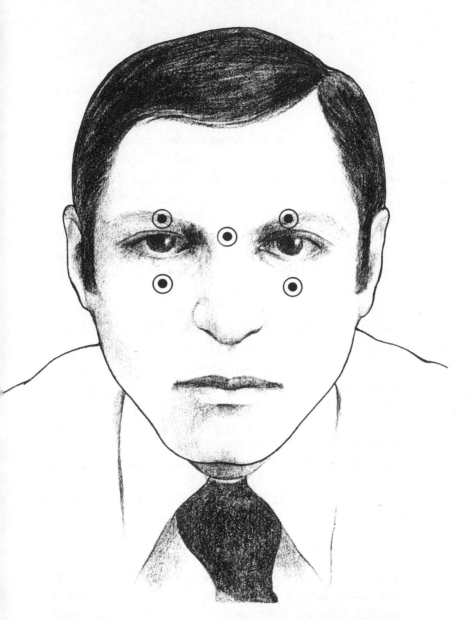

THE SINUS PRESSURE POINTS. *The Sinus 1 pair are directly above the pupils of your eyes, and the Sinus 2 pair are directly below. Nose 1—the only headache pressure point that isn't part of a pair—is centered precisely between your two eyebrows.*

Many things can go wrong in these sinus cavities. A bacterial or viral infection can lead to suppuration, in which the cavity fills with pus. Swelling in infected membranes can close off the passages through which the cavities normally drain, and this generally makes the infection more dangerous and more painful. Among other problems that can affect the sinuses are cysts, polyps, tumors, and allergic edema, or swelling of the sinus lining.

Any of these malfunctions can cause pain in various parts of the head. If you are trying to judge whether a headache is of sinus origin rather than springing from some other cause, here are some of the more common distinguishing symptoms:

Location of pain. In frontal sinus disease, the pain is usually felt behind or above the eyes, sometimes on just one side of the head. The forehead may be tender to the touch.

In ethmoid disease, you are likely to feel pain between the eyes. This pain is not often localized on one side.

When the sphenoid sinuses are involved, the pain is usually deep within the head and may not be easy to distinguish from a migraine headache. In the case of maxillary disease, the pain may be over the back teeth and may spread to the cheeks and the region behind the eyes. It is often localized on one side.

✿　✿　✿

Nature of the pain. A sinus-caused headache generally is constant, rather than throbbing. There may be occasional attacks of sharp, shooting pain through or around the eyes, followed by periods when the pain subsides to a more dull, heavy aching. In frontal sinusitis, some patients notice that the pain seems to begin in midmorning and subside in midafternoon. There may be headaches for several days or a week, followed by a week or two of freedom from pain.

What affects the pain? Sinus headaches often grow sharper when you stoop forward. Sudden jarring of the body, as in running or jumping, may cause spasms of sharp, shooting pain.

Unlike a tension headache, a sinus headache may not respond well to closing the eyes or lying down in a darkened room. In some cases, as a matter of fact, lying down can temporarily increase the pain.

Fever. Some sinus infections are accompanied by a high fever, others by a recurrent, slight fever. This is not true of all sinus problems, however. If the pain is caused by swelling of the sinus linings due to allergy, there may be no fever at all.

Disturbances of smell and taste. Like the common cold, a sinus condition can block the nasal passages. This often leads to anosmia, the loss of the sense of smell. If you lose the sense of smell, you are also likely to lose at least some of your sense of taste. Foods may seem less interesting than they once did. Less commonly, a sinus infection can bring on a condition called parosmia, in which you seem to smell peculiar odors that are not really there.

Nasal discharge. There may be a discharge of clear mucus—a seemingly ordinary "runny nose," as with a cold. The discharge may also contain pus and other material drained from the affected sinus cavity. In this case, the discharged mucus may be thick and whitish.

Swelling and edema. Your face may develop a "puffy" look, particularly around the eyes and the bridge of the nose. The skin may have a blotchy, reddened appearance, and your eyes may seem red and watery. To an untrained observer, in short, you may look as though you are suffering from a chronic cold.

These are some of the signs. I have not listed them here with any thought of encouraging you to diagnose yourself. Self-diagnosis is foolish and unreliable, even for physicians. I have given you this list simply to help you prepare yourself for a visit to your doctor. Go down the list and check off any of the symptoms that you think you have noticed, and then tell your doctor about them. This will give him useful guidance in making his own diagnosis.

In the case of sinus headaches, acupressure may serve a double function. It relieves pain and also may relieve some of the congestion that might be causing or contributing to the pain.

There are many brands of drugs, some sold by prescription and others sold over the counter, that offer to produce the same two results. Let us look briefly at some of those drugs. I would like to convince you that your life will be better—and perhaps will last longer—if you stop taking them.

Many popular cold and sinus remedies—Dristan, Coricidin, Super Anahist, Alka Seltzer Cold Tablets—contain aspirin as a pain reliever. We have already seen some of the dangers in that drug. Other mass-market remedies—Co-Tylenol, Sinutab, Sinarest—contain acetaminophen. This is an analgesic, or pain deadener, that is advertised as lacking some of aspirin's toxic effects and is recommended for people in whom those effects are unusually severe. However, acetaminophen is also toxic in its own way. An overdose can cause liver failure and, in rare cases, even death. Anybody with less than a perfectly healthy liver should be cautious about taking this drug.

Nearly all cold and sinus medicines also contain antihistamines, which are designed to reduce the "runny nose" condition. These often cause drowsiness, which could have lethal effects if you get behind the wheel of a car or operate any other dangerous machine. At best, this drowsiness can affect your work. Many popular sinus drugs include caffeine, a stimulant that is supposed to counteract that drowsy condition. However, the usual dose of thirty milligrams of caffeine is unlikely to have much effect. A cup of coffee contains about one hundred milligrams.

Most of these same medicines contain decongestants. These are designed to constrict swollen blood vessels in the mucous membranes of the nose and sinus cavities. However, the problem is that decongestants do not affect those blood vessels alone. They constrict all the blood vessels in the body. In so doing, they generally raise the blood pressure—which, in some people, can be dangerous.

With auto-acupressure, you can get relief without the hazards. The choice is yours to make.

CHAPTER
10

THE
SINUS
PRESSURE
POINTS

IF YOUR MEDICAL DOCTOR determines that your headaches originate from a sinus condition, then ask his advice about pain relief. In all likelihood he will tell you
that you can use auto-acupressure safely as long as you
follow all of his other directions with care. His aim—
and of course it should be yours too—will be to attack
the underlying problem that is causing the pain. That
process may take some time, for sinus problems do not
always yield to treatment as quickly as the sufferer
might wish. While you are waiting for the doctor's
treatment to take effect, auto-acupressure can help you
control the pain without subjecting yourself to dangerous drugs.

I must warn you that, in using acupressure, there
is potential danger of a different kind. The danger lies
in its remarkable effectiveness. If you find that your
pain is significantly relieved, you may be tempted to
assume your sinus condition has been cured or has
gone away by itself. That is a dangerous assumption,
for it may make you too casual about seeing your doctor regularly. More than many other headache-causing
conditions, sinus infections usually call for frequent
medical checkups and renewals or changes of treatment.
If your doctor requests return visits, do not ignore him.
Follow his advice.

Now let us look at the sinus pressure points. As
with the Group One points, I will begin by telling you
what and where they are, and then I will give you some
special directions on how and in what order to use
them.

WHAT AND WHERE THEY ARE

SINUS 1

Chinese name: *Yu Yao*
Suggested pronunciation: *you-yow*
Translation: Fish Waist
Affected nerve: The supraorbital nerve, which runs above the eye and is connected with a complex of other nerves in the head and face.

How to find it: It lies in the center of your eyebrow, directly above the pupil of your eye when you are looking straight ahead. If you run your thumbnail along your eyebrow, digging in slightly, you will find a small depression at the indicated place. Sinus 1 is in that depression.

As with all the other points, it is important to find exactly the right spot. If you are a fraction of an inch off target, you will merely be pressing on bone and of course will get no significant headache relief. The Sinus 1 point, like the others, has a definitely tender feeling when you are pressing it properly.

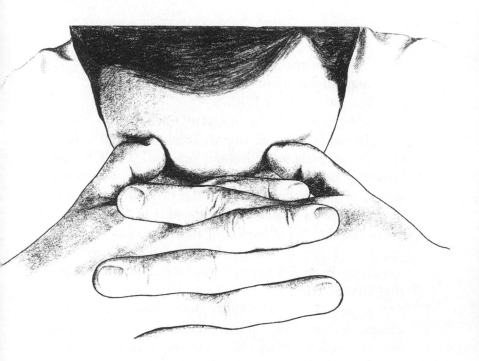

HOW TO PRESS SINUS 1. *As with other paired points on the head, use a hand position that is comfortable and allows you to exert hard pressure. Some prefer to interlace the fingers, as shown. Others put the fingers on the forehead or top of the head.*

SINUS 2

Chinese name: *Szu Pai*
Suggested pronunciation: *sue pie*
Translation: Four Whites
Affected nerve: The infraorbital nerve.

How to find it: It is directly below the pupil of your eye. Put your thumbnail about one and a half finger-breadths below your lower eyelid. The thumbnail should be resting on bone—the top of your cheekbone, or more exactly the lower ridge of your eye socket. Move the thumbnail back and forth beneath your eye pupil until you find a small depression. It will feel something like a tiny notch in the bone. Sinus 2 is within that little notch.

Press inward and slightly downward, not upward toward the eye. You should feel hard resistance from the bone behind the notch. If you find yourself pressing into a soft, fleshy area and displacing your eyeball, you have missed the target. You are too high. On the other hand, if your thumbnail is on the main protuberance of your cheekbone—the rounded portion of it—you are too low. Sinus 2 is in the very rim of the bony eye socket.

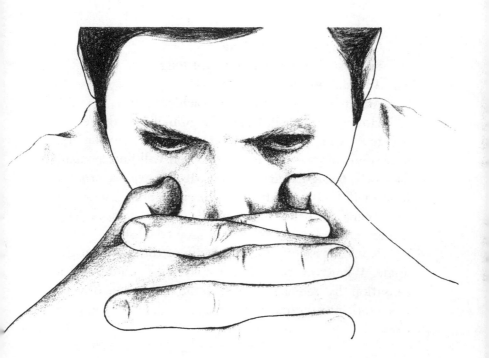

HOW TO PRESS SINUS 2. *The laced-finger position shown is effective for most people. Note that the pressure is directly against the bony ridge—inward and slightly downward. Don't let your thumbnail slide into the soft, fleshy area just below the eye.*

NOSE 1

Chinese name: *Yin Tang*
Suggested pronunciation: *yin tang*
Translation: Seal Hall
Affected nerve: The supratrochlear nerve.

How to find it: Put your thumbnail just above the bridge of your nose, exactly at midpoint between the inner ends of your two eyebrows. You will find a small, flattened, triangular area of bone. If you explore around it you will find two ridges—one on each side. These are the inner ends of the bony ridges over your eyes. The triangular area is formed where they converge.

Nose 1 is exactly in the middle of the flattened triangle. When you press it correctly, you should feel a sensation that seems to spread to the inner parts of your nose and into the passage leading to the back of your throat.

HOW TO USE THEM

GENERAL DIRECTIONS

Use the same pressure technique I have explained under "general directions" for the Group One points. To reiterate briefly, this means using hard pressure with the thumbnail, either steadily or in a rhythmic off-and-on technique, for fifteen to thirty seconds.

The sinus and nose points may need to be stimu-

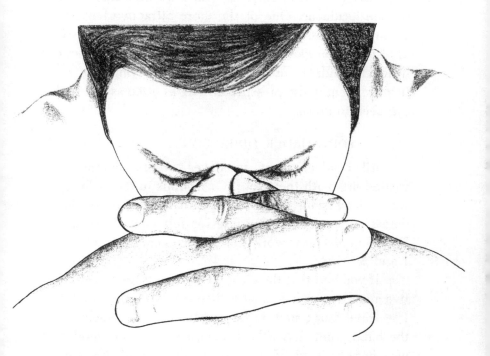

HOW TO PRESS NOSE 1. *Lace the fingers so as to make a single strong unit of the two hands. Use one thumb to reinforce the other, and push the thumbnail in hard. There should be a strong awareness of a "traveling" sensation in the nose and perhaps the throat.*

lated much more often than would be necessary for a tension headache. One of the more attractive features of auto-acupressure, of course, is that you can use it as often as you like with no danger of overdose. If your headache and/or stuffed or runny nose symptoms return frequently, use pressure at will, as often as you feel the need to do so.

POINT-ORDER DIRECTIONS

All headaches, of whatever origin, should be treated first with the Group One points in the ordinary way. Many sinus sufferers find that the Group One points are perfectly adequate for relieving their pain. Try them first. If it works for you, you can ignore Sinus 1 and 2.

If you find that the Group One points are not effective against your headaches, then turn to Sinus 1 and 2. Use Hand 1 or 2 first, however. As you will remember, the hand points have the function of reducing tenderness in your head. If you do not use one of the hand points first, you may find that you are reluctant to apply the necessary hard pressure points on your head.

Use Nose 1 last. The function of this special point will be explained below.

POINT-BY-POINT DIRECTIONS
SINUS 1

Pressure on this point is designed particularly to

relieve congestion in the frontal sinuses, the ones above the eyes. The congestion may be temporarily relieved at the same time as the head pain.

With this point, as with Sinus 2, there is no convenient way to augment thumb leverage by applying opposing force with the fingers. You simply have to push with your thumbs, remembering to keep them bent so as to get the maximum force from thumb and hand muscles.

Most people find it comfortable to clasp the fingers in front of the forehead so as to make a single, strong unit of the two hands. Others prefer to rest the fingertips on the forehead or just behind the hairline, with the hands side by side. Still others find it more effective to put one hand over the other, resting the fingers of the bottom hand flat on the forehead.

Both the Sinus 1 points should be pressed simultaneously, even if your headache seems to be entirely on one side.

SINUS 2

Press this point to relieve congestion in, and pain arising from, the lower sinuses, particularly the maxillary.

Remember, again, to keep your thumbs bent. For some people, this pair of points can be pressed very effectively by clasping the fingers in front of the nose, or by clasping them in such a way that the tip of the nose touches one forefinger. Others find they can generate more force by making the two hands into fists and pushing the two sets of knuckles together below or in front of the nose. As is true of all acupressure points, you will find your own best approach by experimenting. The approach that suits you best will depend on factors such as the relative size of your head and hands, the length of your thumbs, the strength of your hands and wrists.

Like all other paired points, the Sinus 2 pair should be pressed simultaneously. As I have noted before, the apparent or subjective location of any pain sensation is not always a reliable indication of its source. Pain can be referred from a diseased or injured area to some other area quite far away on the body, and this sometimes happens with sinus headaches. Pain on the left often indicates a problem on the left—but not always. It can happen that an infection in the left maxillary sinus, for example, produces pain in the right side of the head. If you press the sinus point on that side only, you may not relieve the pain at all—or, just as frustrating, you may make it "travel" to the other side. Thus, always press both sides.

NOSE 1

This single point, when you press it correctly, is helpful in clearing a stuffed nose and alleviating a runny nose. Pressure on this point, unlike the others, does not act directly to relieve head pain. But it may relieve pain indirectly by helping to clear the nasal passages.

To press this point with good effect, use your strongest hand—your right hand, in other words, if you are right-handed. Put the hand crosswise on your forehead, with the nail of your bent thumb in the Nose 1 triangle and your fingertips against or just above your temple. Push until you feel a sensation of pressure within and behind your nose.

For greater effect, some people find it useful to reinforce the pressing thumb with the fingers or thumb of the other hand.

Let me remind you here that, while the pressure must be forceful on this and all other points, it should *never* be so strong as to break the skin. I mention it here because, unlike the other pressure points, with the exception of Head 1 (the areas just beyond the outer edge of the eye sockets), Nose 1 is really the only point where a blemish would be conspicuous. Nobody wants to walk around wearing the mark of Cain at the top of his nose.

When stimulating a point such as Nose 1, common sense is required. It may be necessary, in order to exert adequate force, for a "Junior Miss" to brace the fingers of the pressing hand against the temple and reinforce the pressing thumb with the other hand, as described. For a "Hercules type" to do this with all his strength would be overzealous.

CHAPTER
11

IF ACUPRESSURE DOESN'T SEEM TO WORK

FOR MOST PEOPLE, the performance of auto-acupressure improves with practice. Each time they use it, they locate the pressure points more surely and press more forcefully. Success brings confidence, which brings more success.

But there are some who have trouble with the technique. I have talked to many patients about their difficulties and helped them analyze the problems involved. In some cases, I have been able to suggest remedies, and in other cases, the patients themselves have told me about tricks that they discovered for themselves. What follows is a list of the more common difficulties I have observed, along with some suggested ways to resolve them. If auto-acupressure is not working as well for you as you expected it would, use this chapter as a troubleshooting checklist. In all likelihood, you will find your problem somewhere in the list.

MISSING THE TARGET

As I have said before, you must locate the pressure points very precisely to be sure you are stimulating nerves with the best possible effect. A seemingly minor error in finding a point could make a major difference.

Recheck the instructions and illustrations in this book if any point seems not to be effective for you. Hunt for the point by probing around the indicated area with your thumbnail. Be alert for that phenomenon of "traveling" sensation; acupressure points are considerably more sensitive than surrounding areas.

One patient told me that he found some of the points more accurately by looking in a mirror. This was particularly true of Sinus 1 and 2. These points are located directly above and below the pupil of the eye when you are looking straight ahead. When he checked himself in a mirror, the patient discovered that he was nearly half an inch off target.

TIMID PRESSURE

When you are applying it well, acupressure causes fifteen to thirty seconds of pain. The pain is by no means intolerable, and it is certainly an excellent bargain when you consider the hours of headache pain from which it can release you. Still, the pressure *must* be forceful enough to hurt somewhat. If it is less forceful, it will unavoidably be less effective.

Some patients gradually increase the pressure as their confidence increases. That usually leads to excellent results. But others appear to go through a reverse cycle. When they first begin applying acupressure, with the memory of their headaches still fresh in their minds, they press willingly and hard. The headaches are relieved. After a few weeks or months, they forget how badly their headaches used to hurt and gradually become less willing to tolerate the short pain of acupressure. They press more and more timidly. The headaches return.

STOPPING TOO SOON

As previously discussed, pressure should be maintained for fifteen to thirty seconds, either steadily or in a rhythmic off-and-on fashion. Talking to patients who had not enjoyed good results, I discovered that many of them were merely guessing at the span of time. When I advised them to time themselves with a watch or clock, most of them reported significant improvement.

Look at a watch or clock now and wait while it counts off thirty seconds. The time span will probably seem longer than you thought it would. Since acupressure does cause some pain, the temptation is to hurry it, cut it short. If you allow yourself to do that, you are unlikely to get full benefit from the technique.

One woman told me that she tried to time herself by counting, "one thousand one, one thousand two . . ." That is supposedly a fairly accurate way to count off seconds. However, she discovered to her own amusement that she was counting much too fast. Particularly toward the end of the thirty-second period, eager to stop pressing, she found herself rushing through the words faster and faster. She finally turned to timing herself by a clock—and discovered, incidentally, that fifteen honest seconds of pressure usually proved enough to relieve her headaches.

A man reported that he found music helpful. He found that the rhythmic off-and-on approach worked best for him. Partly to time himself and partly to distract himself from the pressure, he hummed a catchy tune whose rhythm matched that of his thumbs.

AVOIDING REPEAT TREATMENTS

Just as you may need to take repeated doses of a pain-killing drug, so you may need repeated applications of auto-acupressure if a headache persists or returns. Some patients seem to shy away from repeated treatments. If a headache is not totally relieved after the first treatment on a given day, they become disappointed and give up.

A major advantage of acupressure is that there is no limit to the number of treatments you can give yourself in a day. There are such limits, of course, with all analgesic drugs. Do not be afraid to re-treat yourself if your head continues to ache. And do not expect more from acupressure than it can reasonably be asked to do.

It is not "magic." If a headache is unusually severe or persistent, you may need to repeat the treatments with some frequency. There may be a temporary indentation at the point you have pressed. It may be more sensitive with repetitive stimulation, but that's still a small price to pay for relief from headache pain and freedom from drugs.

PANIC

Another common reason for failure is fear of a returning headache. A patient applies acupressure, finds the headache relieved but still feels some residual pain. Then fear sets in. The patient thinks, "The treatment didn't quite work. I still feel the headache lurking in there somewhere. It will be back in full force if I don't do something." And then, in panic, the patient reaches for the old familiar bottle of pills.

Neither acupressure nor any analgesic drug can guarantee to banish every headache completely and instantly. Regardless of whether you use pressure or pills, you may sometimes get only seventy-five percent relief. If that happens with acupressure, do not panic and turn back to drugs. Remember that the degree of relief given you by acupressure is probably just as great as pills would have given you. It would be a mistake to abandon acupressure just because it has failed to give one hundred percent relief.

QUICK HEADACHE RELIEF
WITHOUT DRUGS

When drugs fail to give complete relief, the usual answer—not always a safe one—is more drugs. When acupressure does not give total relief, the perfectly safe answer is more acupressure. If you feel a residue of discomfort after giving yourself a treatment, simply wait to see if the headache does in fact return to its original severity. If you feel the discomfort increasing, apply pressure again.

This is a good place to remind you that an important touchstone of success in perfecting the technique of auto-acupressure is to strive for the funny-bone feeling. If you feel a tingling sensation, you are on the right spot. If you do not, probe around a few millimeters in one direction or another, or press harder, or press more directly with your thumbnail, or dig deeper *under* the bone and tissue protecting the nerve you are trying to reach and stimulate.

CONDITIONED RESPONSE

Some patients are troubled by pain that is not really there but has previously been experienced. This phenomenon is well known to psychiatrists. If you expect to feel pain in a certain situation, you may feel it even though there is no physical basis for it. When I go to a dentist, for example, he may give me novacaine before starting to work on my tooth. The rational part of my mind tells me that there is no possibility of feeling pain in the anesthetized area. Yet, when he starts to drill, I feel pain.

So it is with some headache sufferers when they first try auto-acupressure. For years they have been taking pills to relieve the pain. They have built up a conditioned response: "If I fail to take pills, my head will hurt." Even though acupressure has had its effect, the headache seems to remain because the sufferer expects it to remain.

Many times, I have pressed on a patient's headache points and have seen the following sequence of events: First, the patient complains about the transient pain related to the acupressure. When I ask if the headache pain is still present, the person says without self-examination, "My head still aches." Then I ask about the relative intensity of the headache. I ask whether it is increased or decreased to any significant degree. Often the patient looks amazed when concentration and self-examination reveal how little pain is really left.

After an acupressure treatment, concentrate momentarily on your headache. Does your head *really* still hurt? Is the pain unchanged or has it diminished? Is there still pain, or has the pain been replaced by a slight residue of discomfort? The rapid disappearance of headache pain is a new and unexpected experience. Allow yourself to acknowledge it.

CHANGING MEDICAL CONDITION

In this book I have emphasized the importance of consulting a medical physician about your headaches. Significant pain anywhere in the body, including the head, is a signal that something is wrong. When your body gives you such a signal, you should go to a medical doctor and let him find out what that "something wrong" is. As we have seen, he may determine that the essential cause of your headaches is something for which no practical treatment is possible—an airborne allergen, for example. In that case, he will advise you simply to treat the symptom of the disease, the pain alone. On the other hand, he may discover that the cause not only is treatable but also dangerous if not treated. In this case, he may suggest that you use acupressure while his treatment is going on. Either way, you should be very sure you know what causes your headaches.

If you have not consulted a physician and you find your headaches persisting or growing worse, it may be that they are caused by some unsuspected, gradually worsening condition, such as hypertension or hypoglycemia. Be particularly alert for headaches that start to recur when you thought you had them under control, or for headaches that seem different in quality, location, or severity than those you used to know. This may indicate that some new medical problem has arisen, or that a once-hidden problem is now beginning to come to light. If this happens, consult your physician immediately. Even if there are no such changes, it is a good general policy for any adult to have a thorough medical checkup at least once a year.

PSYCHOLOGICAL STRESSES

Also, be aware of changes going on in your life that might be contributing to your headaches or making them harder to manage. If you enter a period of unusual tension, worry, or unhappiness, this could increase the severity of headaches and reduce the effectiveness of acupressure or any other pain-relieving method.

One woman patient consulted me recently about just such an experience. She had previously found auto-acupressure almost totally effective in combating headaches. Then, unaccountably, the headaches seemed to grow worse, and acupressure became only about fifty percent effective. After giving her an examination that revealed no new physical problems, I asked her about her personal life. Was she fighting any unusual emotional problems? She said no.

I went on talking to her. Gradually, it developed that she was in fact up against some severe problems, but was doing her best to deny their existence. The problems were in her marriage, and they were growing progressively worse. She felt unable to discuss them with her husband. She felt there was no way to solve them, and because of that, she was fighting to convince herself that the problems did not exist.

Her unconscious mind knew they existed, however, and had progressively increased the headache symptoms until she found herself with a medical reason to go to a doctor. In this way, her unconscious forced her to confront the problems that her conscious mind was denying.

If you have any reason to suspect that unresolved emotional difficulties may in some way be involved with your headaches, a visit to a psychiatrist may turn out to be helpful.

A NEED FOR A HEADACHE

Headaches hurt, but they are "useful" sometimes. They have marvelous power to shield us from problems we would rather not face. They can get us out of responsibilities. They can become a license for putting off unpleasant tasks. They can be a weapon of revenge or a demand for sympathy. Some common ways of using headaches:

"Not now, I've got a headache."

"Stop arguing with me! You're giving me a headache!"

"Look what you've done to me."

"Would you mind meeting Mother at the airport? I've got the most awful . . ."

"Yes, I know I didn't do a very good job, but . . ."

"Would you bring me a cup of tea and a pillow?"

"Don't worry, I'll do it just as soon as I feel up to it."

You must be frank with yourself. If your headaches persist, are you sure it is not because you want them to persist?

CHAPTER

12

YOU CAN
EVEN DO IT
IN PUBLIC

ONE OF THE ADVANTAGES of auto-acupressure is that you can apply it whenever and wherever a headache happens to strike you. You could even apply it, if you wished, while sitting on a stage before an auditorium full of people. It can be done in such a way that nobody will realize you are doing anything unusual.

Headaches, of course, are not respecters of time and place. A headache may strike at any inconvenient time: while you are in the middle of a meeting, a dinner party, a holiday trip. Even if pain-killing pills happen to be available at the time, even if you carry them in your pocket or purse, it is not always possible to take them inconspicuously when you need them. And if you have none at hand, the inconvenience is multiplied. Few things surely irritate a host or hostess more than to hear a guest ask, "Do you have any aspirin in the house?"

Here are some hints on using auto-acupressure when other people are around.

((203   ))

QUICK HEADACHE RELIEF
WITHOUT DRUGS

The hand points can of course be pressed at any time without attracting attention. You can hold your hands under a table, for example. If you are not seated at a table or desk, you can pretend to be merely clasping your hands obscured in your lap. Seated on a certain kind of chair, you can even stimulate hand points with your hands behind your back.

Head 1 (the pair of points near the temples) can be pressed publicly in at least two different ways.

You can press them simultaneously by leaning your elbows on a table or desk, as though leaning your head on your hands. This is a relatively common sitting position. Put your fingers above or against your forehead, with the thumbnails in the Head 1 points. You will look to other people as though you are immersed in thought.

An alternate method is to press the Head 1 points, one at a time, with almost any small object, such as the eraser end of a pencil. Simply put the eraser in the Head 1 point and lean your head against it to generate the necessary pressure. This, too, is a fairly common gesture among people who are sitting and thinking. After treating one point for the needed fifteen to thirty seconds, switch unobtrusively to the other side.

Do not use a sharp object that could injure the skin. It would be exceedingly dangerous to try this trick with the pointed end of a pencil, for example. The object you use should be small enough so that, like your thumbnail, it can apply hard pressure to a defined point on a nerve. But it should *not* be so pointed that it can cut or pierce the skin.

The earpiece of a pair of plastic-framed eyeglasses or sunglasses can sometimes serve for this purpose. In this case, hold the earpiece close to its tip so that there is no chance of breaking it. And, of course, do not try the technique with thin wire frames. These are likely to be too sharp.

Head 2 (the pair of points at the back and base of the skull) can also be pressed easily in public. Simply lean back and clasp your hands behind your head— a very common posture. Once you are in that position, you can put your thumbnails into the Head 2 points and press without attracting attention.

The Head 2 points can also be stimulated in public by pressing with the blunt end of a pen or pencil.

The sinus points are more difficult to press in public. Since these points (including Nose 1) are on the front of the face, pressing them leaves thumbnail marks that may be visible to other people. These marks vanish in a few minutes, but you may prefer not to appear in public while they are visible. My suggestion is that you wait until you have a few minutes of privacy before pressing these points.

However, one way to stimulate Sinus 1 in public is to lean over a table with the hands clasped. Support the bent head by thumbnail pressure directly into the center of each eyebrow. This will leave temporary pressure marks only under the eyebrows.

CHAPTER

13

THE POST-GRADUATE PRESSURE POINT

QUICK HEADACHE RELIEF
WITHOUT DRUGS

YOUR BASIC COURSE in auto-acupressure has now been completed, but there is one more pressure point I want to teach you. Let us call it a postgraduate course, or a bonus technique.

I have saved this chapter until last, partly because this last pressure point is somewhat more difficult to locate precisely than the other headache points and partly because, once you master it, this is one of the most effective techniques of all. Unlike the others, stimulation of this point may need to be used sparingly. The pressure point seems easy to find, but it is not. You may not find it at all until you have had practice with the other points.

In dealing with this point even more than with the others, pay special attention to the odd sensation of nerve stimulation that occurs when you are properly on target. The sensation in all cases seems to travel beyond the single point being pressed. As I have noted, it is like the tingling sensation that travels up your arm when you hit the so-called funny bone in your elbow. The tingling sensation may also travel down to the tip of your little finger. This phenomenon of traveling stimulation is particularly important with the last pressure point I am about to deal with. If you are not *exactly* on target, you will notice only a sensation of pain at the point itself. You may need to do a considerable amount of experimenting before you feel the sensation radiating beyond the point.

I call this point *Hand 3*. It differs from all the other points in one respect: Instead of pressing with a thumbnail, you *pinch* it between a thumbnail and fingernail.

Like the other two hand points, this one serves to lessen tenderness in the head, so that you can press the head points without causing yourself too much pain. In many people, once they master it, Hand 3 is the most effective of all the hand points, especially for *sinus problems*. When properly located and properly pinched, it sometimes gives complete headache relief all by itself. In any case, I suggest it as an alternate starting routine for patients who find the other two hand points too tender or who, for some reason, do not get adequate head pain relief from the other two. After you have learned to find Hand 3, experiment with it the next few times you have a headache. If you find that it works better for you than Hand 1 and 2, use it instead of them, or in conjunction with them.

As I noted before, unlike all the other points described in this book, stimulation of the pinch point may need to be done sparingly. A persistent numbness or tingling may result for a while after stimulation of this point. These sensations may be in the little finger below the pinch point that was stimulated, or may be in the elbow area above it. Do *not* restimulate the pinch point until after the sensations of numbness or tingling have entirely vanished.

HAND 3: THE PINCH POINT

Chinese name: *Hou Hsi*
Suggested pronunciation: *hoo see*
Translation: Back Stream
Affected nerves: Branches of the ulnar nerve.

How to find and pinch it: First hold either hand out, palm up. Start to close your hand into a fist. As your palm starts to fold, notice the long crease that begins under your little finger and runs all, or nearly all, the way across the palm toward the base of the index finger. Continue to close your hand until you end with a tightly clenched fist. Notice that the end of the crease is still visible below the little finger. Where the crease ends, a triangular fold of flesh protrudes from the edge of your hand.

The Postgraduate Pressure Point

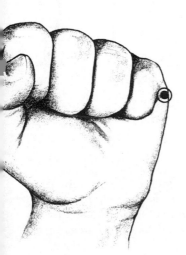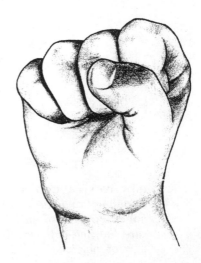

HOW TO FIND THE PINCH POINT. *The point is on that little pyr-amid-shaped fold of flesh that sticks out at the base of your little finger when you make a fist. The nerve you are looking for is at the base of the pyramid, hard up against the bone. Note visible crease on right hand below little finger.*

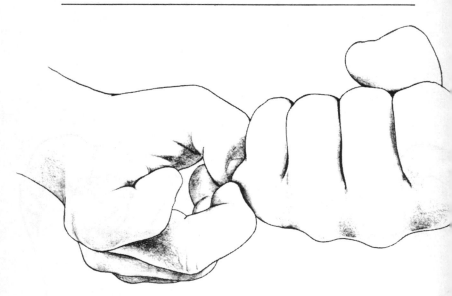

HOW TO STIMULATE THE PINCH POINT—LEFT HAND. *Use the thumbnail and the nail of the middle finger, not the index finger. Pinch hard, into the flesh and against the bone. Make sure the two nails are directly opposed like the blades of a pair of pincers.*

The pinch point, Hand 3, is within that small triangular protuberance. Grasp it between the nails of your thumb and *middle* finger, with your thumb on the palm side and the finger on the back. Note that the "pincers" is at right angles to the palm, not parallel to it. It is important to use the middle finger, rather than the index finger, for the nerve is stimulated most effectively when the two nails are directly opposed like the blades of a pair of pincers. Most people's hands

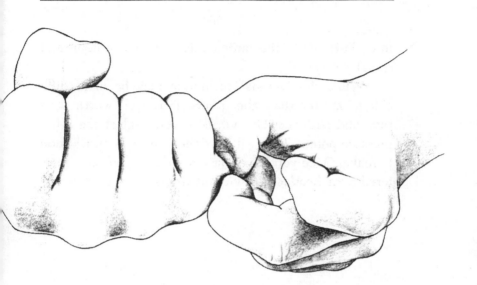

HOW TO STIMULATE THE PINCH POINT—RIGHT HAND. *Experiment on both hands until you feel the sensation "traveling." Again, apply sufficient pressure to produce a reasonably prolonged tingling sensation, not less than ten seconds, not more than thirty.*

are so shaped that it is difficult to get good opposition between the thumbnail and the index fingernail.

Push the two nails inward against the bone at the edge of your hand and sharply pinch the fleshy triangle. When you are on target, you should feel a sensation traveling down the edge or back of your hand toward the wrist. If you feel no sensation, move the "pincers" away from the bone a millimeter or two. The sensation, when you feel it, is traveling along branches of the ulnar nerve—which, as we noted before, links with the autonomic nervous system and spinal cord at the neck.

While this "bonus" technique may be more difficult to master than the others, it is well worth your time and patience. Do not, however, neglect the other pressure points. They all have their special contribution to make. Once you have mastered them, you have mastered your headaches, without drugs.

AFTERWORD

I HAVE NOW presented what you need to know about how and when to achieve relief from headache pain with auto-acupressure. The rest is up to you.

"A fine tool is nothing except in a skilled hand," says a Chinese proverb. And so it is with auto-acupressure. It is a fine tool. It will serve you well if you learn when to use it and how to use it skillfully.

To become adept at any skill requires knowledge and practice. Acupressure for headache relief is not an exceptionally difficult skill, but it does need patience and effort if it is to be learned well. I hope you will give it that patience and effort.

If you do, the rewards you gain will last the rest of your life. And once you have mastered the technique, be a friend to your friends and to your family. Tell them about relieving pain without drugs. Encourage them to obtain their physicians' recommendations about including pain-relief from headaches with auto-acupressure as part of a comprehensive medical treatment program. And the next time you find yourself reaching for the pain medicine bottle, remember that you have a drug-free alternative—auto-acupressure.

INDEX

accessory points, 132
  first pressed, 151-152
acetaminophen, 171
acetylsalicylic acid, 20
acupressure, auto-acupressure:
  vs. acupuncture, 22, 39
  for common headaches, 92, 127-161
  for electroshock headaches, 50
  inconspicuous, 38, 203-205
  pressure required for, 148, 149-151, 190-191
  repeated treatments of, 23, 180-182, 192-193, 194, 209
  resolving difficulties with, 189-199
  serious disease and, 93
  for sinus headaches, 92-93, 175-185, 209
  skepticism toward, 24-26, 35-36
  techniques of, 147-161, 180-185, 210-214
  thumbnails used in, see thumbnails
  timing of, 148, 191-192
acupuncture, 22, 45-46
  author's experience with, 47-49
  differing systems of, 62
  faddish aspects of, 24-25, 57-59
  history of, in East, 60-63
  history of, in West, 56-59
  Shiatsu vs., 39-40
  in surgery, 58, 65

airborne allergens, 76, 93-94, 196
alcohol, 87, 115, 116, 120
Alice's Adventures in Wonderland, 98
allergies, 76, 90, 113
  to drugs, 122, 123
  sinuses and, 165, 168, 169
American Psychiatric Association, California meeting of (1975), 26-27
Anacin, 20, 23
analgesia, from acupuncture, 59
anatomical snuffbox, 142
anesthesia, vs. analgesia, 58-59
angina pectoris, 61
Annette, J. (case history), 85-89, 91, 95, 116, 122
anosmia, 169-170
anoxia, 102
antihistamines, 171-172
arteries:
  dilation of, 76, 83, 101, 115
  thickening of, 114
aspirin, 20, 21, 23, 27, 55, 60, 153, 171
associative headaches, 90
auditory hallucinations, 117
aura, as headache warning, 81, 101-102, 107

barbiturates, 21
barefoot doctors, in China, 64
biofeedback, 99-100
birth-control pills, 97

Index

finger needle, 49
Fred C. (case history), 38-39, 40, 41-42
frontal sinuses, 166, 168, 183

gangrene, 102
gastric irritation, aspirin and, 21
general-system diseases, 123
George R. (case history), 71-77, 86, 87, 89, 91, 94, 113
grand mal seizures, 111
Grant, Ulysses S., 98

hallucinations, 101, 117
Hand 1, 138-140, 151, 182, 204, 209
 pregnancy and, 152-153
 technique for pressing, 154-155
hands, warming of, 99-100
Hand 2, 140-143, 151, 182, 204, 209
 pregnancy and, 152-153
 technique for pressing, 156-157
Hand 3, 208-214
headaches:
 associative vs. chronic, 90
 criteria for treatment of, 99, 103
 diagnosis and classification of, 69, 70, 89-93, 107-108
 as electroshock side effect, 50
 faked vs. real, 75
 family history and, 96-97, 119
 location of, 114, 168
 nature of pain of, 115, 169
 onset history of, 113
 other factors in, 121-123
 personality and, 98, 119-121
 precipitating factors in, 116
 progression of, 114
 questions about, 112-123
 suffering in, 19-20, 21-22, 32, 69-70
 symptoms associated with, 117
 time patterns of, 115-116

worsening or relief of, 118-119
head injuries, 121
Head 1, 133-136, 152, 185
 inconspicuous pressing of, 204-205
 technique for pressing, 158
Head 2, 136-137, 152
 inconspicuous pressing of, 205
 technique for pressing, 160-161
heart muscle damage, 102
hematomas, 121
high blood pressure, see hypertension
histamine, 83
histamine cephalgia, 27, 83-84, 92
 symptoms of, 83, 115, 117
Ho Ku, see Hand 1
hormonal changes, 97
Hou Hsi, see Hand 3
hunger headaches, 110, 122
hypalgesia, 59, 65
hypertension, 99, 114, 117, 119, 196
hypoglycemia, 31, 110, 116, 118, 122, 196

intracranial pressure, 118

Jeanette T. (case history), 36-38, 41, 42

Kurland, Howard D.:
 empirical-eclectic approach to medicine of, 55-56
 herniated disk problem of, 46-49

letdown migraines, 76-77, 116
Lieh Chueh, see Hand 2
life-styles, change of, 94
Linda W. (case history), 108-112, 116
liver, acetaminophen and, 171
low blood sugar, see hypoglycemia

Index

LSD, 101
lumbago, 57

main points, 132
Mao Tse-tung, 64
masseurs, as Shiatsu practitioners, 39-40
maxillary sinuses, 166, 168, 183
medicine:
    ancient Oriental concepts of, 56, 63
    empiricism in, 55
    modern American, 65
    in modern China, 64
medicines, derived from plants, 65
meningitis, 113
meningoencephalitis, 113
menopause, 97
menstruation, 97
methysergide maleate tablets (Sansert), 100-101
migraines, 21, 23, 27, 36, 69, 90, 93
    biofeedback for, 99-100
    vs. histamine cephalgia, 88
    as inheritable, 96-97, 119
    letdown, 76-77
    personality and, 98
    prevention of, 100-101
    symptoms of, 101-102, 107, 113, 114, 117, 118
mirror, to locate points, 190
monosodium glutamate, 88-89
mothering, pills and, 37
muscle-contraction headaches, see tension headaches
myocardial infarction, 102

narcotics, 50, 102-103
nasal discharge, 170
National Institute of Health, 59
nausea, 102, 117
needles, acupuncture and, 22, 39, 40, 48, 57, 63

nervous systems:
    acupuncture and, 60
    imbalance in, 76, 90, 130
neuralgia, 117
New York State Board for Medicine, 59
New York State Commission on Acupuncture, 60
Nixon, Richard M., China trip of (1972), 57, 64
Northwestern University Medical School, 26
Nose 1, 180, 182, 205
    technique for pressing, 184-185

off-and-on pressure, 148-149, 191
olfactory hallucinations, 117
oral contraceptives, 97
organically caused headaches, 91
Osler, Sir William, 57
overdose deaths, 21

pain:
    acupressure relief of, explained, 128-130, 148
    as conditioned response, 194-195
    vs. drug danger, 21-22, 27, 103
    nature of, 115, 169
    referred, 61, 184
paramedical practitioners, in China, 64
paranasal sinuses, 165-168
parosmia, 170
peptic ulceration, aspirin and, 21
phenacetin, 21
physical examinations:
    ancient Chinese, 61-62
    importance of, 107-108, 123, 196-197
physical exertion, as headache cure, 85
pill-taking, in our society, 35-37
pilots, grand mal seizures of, 111
pinch point (Hand 3), 208-214

((223))